THE FACE BOOK

THE FACE BOOK

The Pros and Cons
of Facial Plastic Surgery

**Prepared by the
American Academy of
Facial Plastic and
Reconstructive Surgery**

ACROPOLIS BOOKS LTD.
WASHINGTON, D.C.

ACROPOLIS BOOKS, LTD.
Alphons J. Hackl, Publisher
Colortone Building, 2400 17th St., N.W.
Washington, D.C. 20009

Attention: Schools and Corporations
ACROPOLIS books are available at quantity discounts with bulk purchase for educational, business, or sales promotional use. For information, please write to: SPECIAL SALES DEPARTMENT, ACROPOLIS BOOKS, LTD., 2400 17th St., N.W., WASHINGTON, D.C. 20009.

Are there Acropolis books you want but cannot find in your local stores?
You can get any Acropolis book title in print. Simply send title and retail price. Be sure to add postage and handling: $2.25 for orders up to $15.00; $3.00 for orders from $15.01 to $30.00; $3.75 for orders over $100.00. District of Columbia residents add applicable sales tax. Enclose check or money order only, no cash please, to:

ACROPOLIS BOOKS LTD.
2400 17th St., N.W.
WASHINGTON, D.C. 20009

The information in this book is believed to be accurate and to reflect the current state of medical science. However, new techniques are constantly being developed in facial plastic surgery. Moreover, each patient's care necessarily requires individual attention. Therefore, this book does not offer medical advice and is not a medical treatise. Patients contemplating facial plastic surgery should not rely on this book for advice but should consult a facial plastic surgeon. All surgery is serious and can involve complications. To the extent the facial plastic surgeon's advice differs from anything stated in this book, the patient should follow the surgeon's directions.

Library of Congress Cataloging-in-Publication Data
The face book: the pros and cons of facial plastic surgery/prepared by the American Academy of Facial Plastic and Reconstructive Surgery.
     p. cm.
   ISBN 0-87491-914-2: $19.95
   1. Surgery, Plastic-Popular works. I. American Academy of Facial Plastic and Reconstructive Surgery.
RD119.F3 1988
617'. 520592-dc19
88-14383 CIP

Acknowledgments

The American Academy of Facial Plastic and Reconstructive Surgery (AAFPRS) was founded almost 25 years ago with education as its primary mission. While most of its programming has been dedicated to the continuing education needs of facial plastic surgeons, the Academy also has been concerned with keeping the public abreast of advances in facial plastic surgery so that informed consumers could make wise choices about whether to have this surgery and, if so, how to choose a facial plastic surgeon.

In a real sense, then, The Face Book would not have been possible without the work of the more than 3,100 facial plastic surgeons who comprise the AAFPRS. It is this group, collectively, that has developed and refined our specialty in order to bring to patients the techniques that are discussed in this book and, in so doing, to help them feel more confident and happier about themselves. The Academy gratefully acknowledges the work of the full membership and extends special thanks to those facial plastic surgeons who made specific contributions of their time, knowledge, and experience to produce this book.

Foremost thanks go to the AAFPRS Face Book Editorial Board, who worked many hours in the development, writing, and review of this book: E. Gaylon McCollough, M.D., chairman; Ferdinand F. Becker, Jr., M.D.; G. Jan Beekhuis, M.D.; John R. Hilger, M.D.; Frank M. Kamer, M.D.; Norman J. Pastorek, M.D.; Robert L. Simons, M.D.; and J. Regan Thomas, M.D.

Dr. Beekhuis merits special thanks for his contribution of much written material for large sections of this book.

For sharing their papers and insights, thanks go to Jack R. Anderson, M.D.; Saul Asken, M.D.; Louis E. Costa, M.D.; Steven M. Denenberg, M.D.; Nabil Fuleihan, M.D.; Richard W. Fleming, M.D.; Gregory S. Keller, M.D.; Russell W. H. Kridel, M.D.; Devinder S. Mangat, M.D.; Daniel E. Rousso, M.D.; and Larry D. Schoenrock, M.D.

All of these surgeons are leaders in the field of facial plastic surgery, and it is a testament to their surgical skills that their patients vied for the opportunity to tell how their surgery affected their lives.

Thanks also to those who, with their patients' permission, contributed "before and after" photographs that enabled us to illustrate the dramatic improvements that facial plastic surgery makes for many patients. A separate table of illustrations indicating the patients and surgeons follows the table of contents.

We owe a special debt to the patients who provided accounts of their experiences. Most people who have had facial plastic surgery are happy to talk about it. In most cases, the patients' own names have been used with their permission. In some cases, the names have been changed to protect confidentiality. In some other cases, to avoid any intrusion into privacy, the facts of several surgeries have been combined into a description that, the Academy believes, accurately reflects typical experiences.

The Academy gratefully acknowledges Paul Forbes and his associates at the Forbes Group and AAFPRS attorney Thomas Rhodes for their contributions.

Finally, but certainly not least of all, we extend special thanks to the editorial team at the Business Service Network, especially Manager Susan Hill Rozynek, Senior Editor Debbie Demmon-Berger, Associate Editors Angela Martin and Fran Cohen Wickham, and Senior Designer Tamara Strickhouser. The Face Book would not have been possible without their unique ability to translate the insights, experiences, and writing of many facial plastic surgeons into seamless prose in a timely manner.

We hope this book gives you some understanding of our members' untiring dedication to making the highest possible quality of facial plastic surgery available to the public. If you are interested in learning more about facial plastic surgery or receiving the names of AAFPRS fellows in your area who participate in the Facial Plastic Surgery Information Service, please feel free to call 800-332-FACE (U.S.), 800-523-FACE (Canada), or 842-4500 (District of Columbia).

Lee VanBremen, Ph.D.
Executive Vice President, AAFPRS

Contents

Table of Illustrations

Partial photo research by Imagefinders, Inc.

The Wonder of Facial Plastic Surgery

WITH HER 50TH BIRTHDAY APPROACHING, Patricia Rile looked older than she felt. As the owner of an upscale women's apparel shop on the West Coast, in business to help women look good, she admits she likes to look sharp.

"It was a cosmetic change," she says of her facelift surgery. "Women change cosmetics constantly. Why not start with the basics, the face itself?"

Why not, indeed? Although facial plastic surgery (plastic surgery of the head and neck) is by no means for everyone, more than two million people—men as well as women, young people as well as the elderly—undergo facial surgery each year. For several reasons that figure is expected to rise.

A contributing factor is medical advances, which in recent years have made commonplace facial improvements that simply were not possible a mere 10 years ago. Laser beams today vaporize skin cancers, lesions, and lumpy scar tissue. Various combinations of synthetic and natural materials replace bone and soft tissue destroyed by cancer. Plastic balloons stretch hair-bearing scalp into balding areas, and injectable materials fill wrinkles and old scars left by acne or chicken pox. Results for many procedures are longer lasting and more natural looking than ever before. No wonder public interest escalates with every announcement of new technology or refinement in surgical procedures.

"I believe that life is too short to stay locked up behind a face you don't like," says a facial plastic surgeon from Birmingham, Mich., who has taken his own advice. "I myself now sport a rejuvenated face, and I certainly don't regret my choice. Through the marvel of facial plastic surgery, you can put your best face forward—making the most of what you have."

This surgeon's view is shared by many. Looking good is something our youth-oriented society demands. More important, it is something that makes us feel better, more self-confident, more in control of our own lives. It is the goal of our endless fitness programs, grooming regimens, and diets—just because it makes us feel better. And it is the goal of facial plastic surgery, a specialty that recently has come of age. This is the surgical specialty that, by repositioning tissue, often can lift the spirits of people with premature signs of aging, unsightly birth defects, and deformities caused by illness or accident.

Since facial plastic surgery today offers such a wide range of help, it is appreciated by a far broader spectrum of people than ever before. For example, a facial plastic surgeon in Santa Barbara, Calif., has used laser technology to treat birthmarks in the head and neck area of nearly 50 children. "The fact that lasers appear to be safe for use on children is one of the most exciting aspects of our work," he says.

Another facial plastic surgeon from St. Louis, Mo., performs reconstructive surgery on trauma victims. He tells of a young construction worker whose forehead was flattened in a 44-foot fall, but who managed to walk to the emergency room before passing into a deep coma. With the skilled use of the best modern science has to offer, the surgeon restored the young man to normal function and appearance.

Improving on Mother Nature

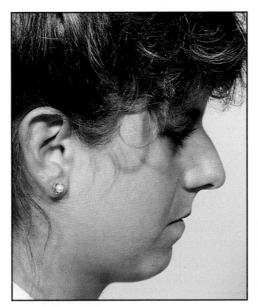 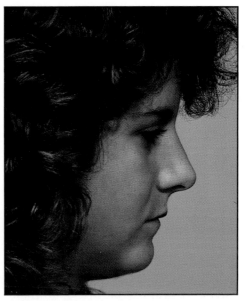

Nasal surgery combined with a chin implant can improve the profile. See chapter 12.

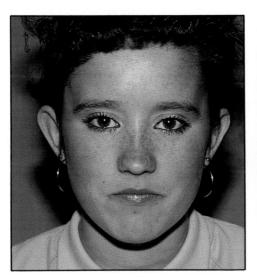 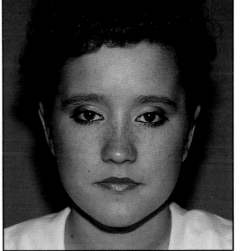

Pinning back protruding ears can reduce a young person's self-consciousness. See chapter 10.

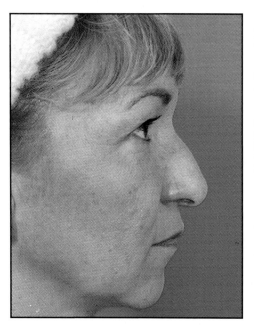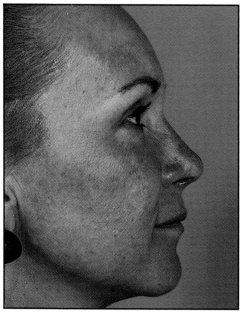

A chin implant, along with nasal and upper eyelid surgery, can produce pleasing results. See chapter 12.

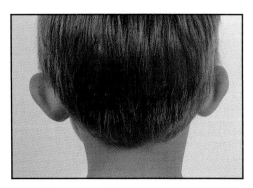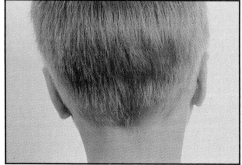

Protruding ears are best corrected at an early age when cartilage is soft. See chapter 10.

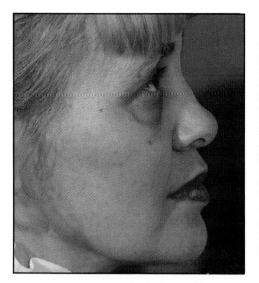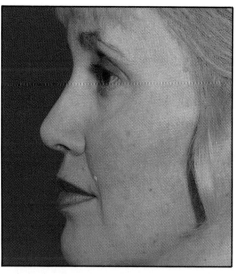

Lower eyelid surgery can be combined with nasal surgery to produce a more youthful appearance. See chapter 11.

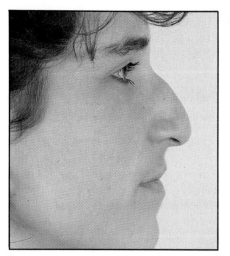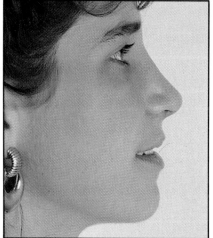

While not usually done on very young children, nasal surgery is a good choice for young people in their mid-teens or older.

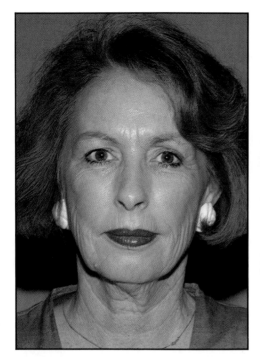
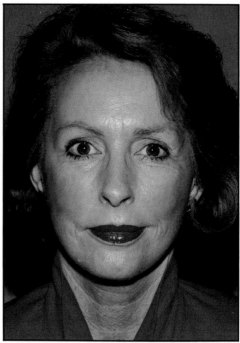

Maye Keao is happy with her facelift, upper and lower eyelid surgery, and chin augmentation. See chapter 8.

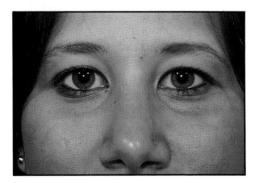
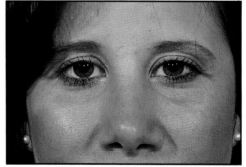

Droopy eyelids can be hereditary. The condition may be improved with facial plastic surgery. See chapter 11.

Still another facial plastic surgeon in Miami Beach, Fla., reports that patients with breathing problems as often as not ask him to improve the appearance of their noses as long as he is operating.

Improving on Mother Nature

As deeply valued as reconstructive work is, the surgical procedures that simply improve appearance get the most coverage in newspaper and magazine articles and on television talk shows. Whether it is performed to lessen signs of aging or improve on Mother Nature, this type of surgery also has its value.

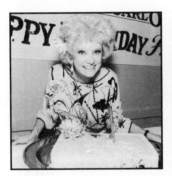 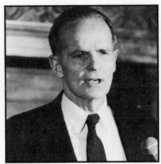 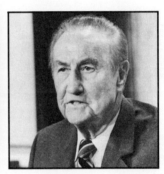

With her much publicized facelift, Phyllis Diller (left) brought facial plastic surgery out of the closet. Politicians William Proxmire (center) and Strom Thurmond added to the respectability of facial plastic surgery when they had hair replacement surgery.

''When I address a community group or lecture at a medical convention, I sometimes hear the comment that purely cosmetic surgery is frivolous or pretentious,'' says the facial plastic surgeon from Birmingham, Mich. ''But it is an invaluable service to those patients who exercise their option to squeeze more bounty from nature's stingy hand. It is important to those people who feel that they need it. And it is not the surgeon's domain to analyze their good reasons for requesting surgical improvement if it is obvious that their complaints match reality.''

People in the public eye have long acknowledged the importance of appearance. Phyllis Diller was perhaps the first public figure to step out of the closet with her facelift and, by so doing, to add to the respectability

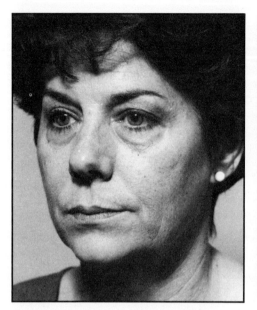 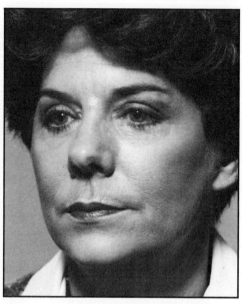

Patricia Rile before and after surgery

of facial plastic surgery. While film and TV stars may still be reluctant to attribute their youthful good looks to facial plastic surgery, more and more ordinary people—not people who are undistinguished, but certainly individuals whose occupations are not necessarily tied to their looks—are consulting facial plastic surgeons.

Patricia Rile at first planned only to have something done about her eyelids. But she changed her mind and decided to go with the whole facelift after her surgeon "pulled my face a little and showed me what it might look like after surgery. He also showed me where my jawline had dropped. I hadn't even noticed I had lost my jawline."

The surgery was a resounding success. Ten days after the facelift was performed, Rile stood up at a fashion show where she was serving as commentator and announced it to the audience. Everyone applauded.

Men, too, are discovering the benefits of improving on nature. Male patients, nearly half of them under 40, account for more than 30 percent of the facial plastic surgery operations performed in this country. "About the only men we used to see were actors,'' says one Beverly Hills facial plastic surgeon. ''Now we see teachers, electrical engineers, and lawyers.''

No longer put off by what used to be considered feminine vanity, men are learning that facial plastic surgery helps project the right image on the job. ''Bags under the eyes can make you look slovenly, even dissolute,'' comments one trial lawyer. ''That isn't going to help before a jury.''

Neither is a receding chin going to project an authoritative aura in the board room. Eyelid surgery and chin implants are sensible options, men are finding.

Those who have had facial plastic surgery, a survey recently revealed, say they would do it again, while those who have not had it cite its reportedly high cost as a drawback. Yet facial plastic surgery today is not just for the rich. More than 50 percent of facial plastic surgery patients earn less than $25,000 a year. Most procedures cost little more than a good health club membership and considerably less than a very bottom-of-the-line new car. And the investment in facial plastic surgery lasts a lot longer.

Psychologists Approve

A recent research project points out how important we perceive appearance to be in the workplace. The experiment involved two groups of job applicants. Makeup was applied to the members of each group prior to their job interviews. One group was told that the makeup was being used to give them an unattractive facial scar. Even though that was not true—the makeup was the same for both groups—because one set of job applicants believed they had scars on their faces, they came away from the interviews convinced that the interviewers had been put off by the scars. The other group of applicants completed their interviews in a far more confident and self-assured manner.

Researchers also have studied just how important physical attractiveness is in male/female relationships. An experiment was conducted in which panel members viewed patients' photographs taken both before and after facial plastic surgery. Those seen after surgery were deemed to have more desirable personalities, to be better potential marriage partners, and to have happier lives than those viewed before surgery. Whether or not we like this emphasis on appearance, it exists, and it may not be all bad.

The point of looking your best, says psychologist Dr. Joyce Brothers, is to be able to forget about yourself and still exude self-confidence. "When you look good and feel great, people treat you as if you're special," she explains. "Your appearance sends signals to others about who you are, how you feel, even about your values and aspirations. When people treat you as if you are intelligent and friendly, you behave that way, and that starts an upward spiral of success."

Abigail Van Buren (Dear Abby) agrees. Looking good is a personal gift to oneself, not a narcissistic indulgence, she says. She is backed by expert psychiatric consultants, all of whom regard a little vanity as a good thing. Attention to one's looks is a sign of self-esteem, just as lack of interest in grooming and outer appearance is an early sign of depression.

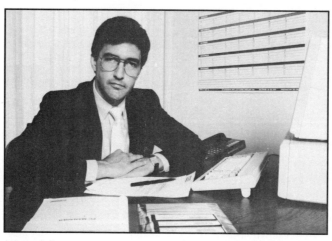

More and more men are turning to facial plastic surgery to help them maintain an executive image.

Dr. Edward Stainbrook, professor emeritus of psychiatry and behavioral science at the University of Southern California's School of Medicine, sees a direct link between the resurgent national interest in healthy bodies and the rise in popularity of facial plastic surgery.

"If you look at the whole social and cultural trend over the last 30 or 40 years, it's moving toward fitness and wellness. There is much less guilt about altering the body. To be physically well means to be physically attractive. And this affects people's willingness to use facial plastic surgery."

This link between health and appearance may well be why most people considering facial plastic surgery have very realistic expectations, according to a recent study. They desire:

- to have a tidy appearance,
- to escape being regarded as different,
- to have the normal physical endowments for the group to which they belong,
- to re-establish a previously satisfactory appearance, or
- to avoid being discounted as a useful member of society on the basis of their age.

Those people who embark on facial plastic surgery with such healthy attitudes often come away not only looking better, but feeling good. "The physical transformation of surgery often is the catalyst that sparks renewed zest for living," says the facial plastic surgeon from Birmingham, Mich. "And this secondary benefit sometimes is far more striking than the anatomical change."

Not for Everyone

Relatively few people harbor unrealistic expectations that facial plastic surgery can totally change their looks and lives. Yet facial plastic surgeons are concerned that the overwhelming message from the media is that this surgery is for everyone. For the record, a new face will not guarantee success on the job or the dating circuit. It will not make people like you more or help a faltering marriage. What it may do is simply make you look better, healthier, and more vibrant.

"When a patient expects facial plastic surgery to solve problems in his or her life, the results are almost doomed to failure," according to the surgeon from Michigan. "Or worse is the case when it's not the patient who wants surgery, but the mother because she thinks the daughter will be more popular after nose reduction surgery."

Some people are unconsciously so comfortable with a facial feature—even one they think they do not like—that a new one, even if cosmetically more attractive, can appear unattractive or "wrong" to them.

Of course, even properly motivated patients may not benefit from facial plastic surgery if they have certain physical traits. Some skin types, for instance, scar too easily to make surgery worthwhile. Likewise, a history of abnormal bleeding is a clear contraindication for this or any elective surgery.

Additionally, a certain amount of risk accompanies any surgical procedure, no matter how healthy the patient or skilled the surgeon. This is surgery, after all, and complications can arise.

Nothing to Hide

Still, for those who want facial plastic surgery, it is an option worth exploring—and it is no longer something to hide. Facelift patients only a decade or two ago used to disappear on a vacation and, when they had returned, persuasively fended off compliments and questions with tales of "a wonderful health spa." Today's patients are totally without guile, far more likely to walk around with nose splints or sunglasses that barely hide facial bruises while the healing process is under way.

Today's patients also are educated consumers. They know that facial plastic surgery has nothing to do with the use of plastic materials, although synthetic implants sometimes are used in certain procedures. The word plastic is derived from the Greek word plastikos, which means "to mold." Facial plastic surgery includes many procedures that basically involve the repositioning of tissue to restore or improve both function and appearance.

It is recorded that more than 3,000 years ago, in India, some of the first nose reconstructions were performed. The procedure was performed

Facial Plastic Surgery Terminology

The actual terminology of facial plastic surgery procedures can be a medical education in itself. To sound more savvy, here is what you need to know:

- *Facial plastic surgeon*—A specialist whose practice is limited primarily to plastic and reconstructive surgery of the face, nose, head, and neck.
- *Rhytidectomy or Rhytidoplasty*—Both simply mean facelift, the removal of excess skin and the tightening of sagging muscles and connective tissue in the face and neck.
- *Rhinoplasty*—A procedure used to change the width, size, and/or shape of the nose.
- *Blepharoplasty*—The removal of excess fat or skin from the upper and/or lower eyelids.
- *Mentoplasty*—Otherwise known as chin augmentation, this procedure involves building up the chin, often using an implant or the patient's own bone.
- *Submental lipectomy*—Surgery to eliminate a double chin.
- *Dermabrasion*—Facial sanding or the use of an abrasive material to buff off the top layers of skin, removing fine facial wrinkles and/or acne scars.
- *Chemabrasion or chemical peel*—Use of a diluted acid on the face, which causes the top layers of skin to slough off, producing smoother, more youthful skin.
- *Otoplasty*—Reshaping the cartilage of protruding ears.
- *Liposuction*—The vacuuming or suctioning of unwanted fat.
- *Scalp flaps*—A repositioning of hair-bearing skin to address baldness.

on criminals whose noses had been cut off as punishment. John Orlando Roe, an otolaryngologist-head and neck surgeon from Rochester, N.Y., was the first facial plastic surgeon in this country. Roe reported the first aesthetic rhinoplasty in 1887. In this century, facial plastic surgery really begins during World War I, when surgeons from many specialties, notably Sir Harold Gillies in England, another renowned otolaryngologist-head and neck surgeon, cooperated to reconstruct the shattered faces of countless young soldiers. One man in particular, Jacques Joseph of Berlin, did much to advance the art of rhinoplasty and facial plastic surgery. He was the first physician to record the now accepted, compassionate philosophy that an abnormal appearance can scar the personality. Dr. Joseph trained many surgeons from all over the world, and one of them, Samuel Foman of New York, brought back his ideas and taught them to facial plastic surgeons in the United States. Since then, of course, innumerable refinements have been made.

Most Popular Procedures

Today, nose reconstruction or rhinoplasty is the most popular facial plastic surgery procedure. More than 500,000 people a year contact facial plastic surgeons in search of a more aesthetically pleasing nose. Scarring is minimal, since the surgery often is done through the nostrils, and overall inconveniences are relatively minor.

Upper and lower eyelid tucks are becoming more popular, especially among men who hold positions in which eye contact is necessary. Upper eyelid surgery usually lasts about 10 years, while lower-lid surgery tends to be more permanent. A separate procedure can remove or minimize laugh lines and crow's feet.

Facelifts are what come to most people's minds when they think of facial plastic surgery, and women and men are having them done at increasingly earlier ages. A good starting point, some surgeons say, is in the late 30s and early 40s when facial skin is still supple. Because the skin of the face and neck continues to age after a facelift, subsequent touchups may be needed; however, the overall aging effect will be minimized. If, for example, the patient is 46 years old and undergoes successful facelift surgery, when that individual is 56, he or she may look only about 48 or so.

This Book is for You

''I think the nicest compliment I've had is that nobody has noticed my surgery,'' comments Patricia Rile. ''Nobody has said, 'Gee, what did you do to your face?' I get other comments, like 'You look pretty today.' I've had compliments about my eyes, people telling me I have pretty eyes. I hadn't heard anything like that in years.''

Patricia Rile can make that statement because she learned all she could about facial plastic surgery and then spent the time needed to find a highly qualified and experienced facial plastic surgeon. In this book, we are going to help you explore these same areas.

''I believe knowledge provides insight; insight aids choice,'' says the surgeon from Michigan. ''It is your right as a patient to expect a full disclosure of all the facts that pertain to your health and well-being—as well as any proposed surgery.''

This book is designed to fill this need, although its scope is limited. It is intended to supplement the information any given doctor will relay to his patients. Yet no doctor has the time to sit down and give you this amount of information during a single consultation. That is why it is paramount for your own protection and essential for your decision-making process to become better informed regarding your options in the field of facial plastic surgery.

We will start this educational journey with some simple charts and narrative that will help you analyze your face in much the same way a facial plastic surgeon would. In part I, you will see how your face measures up to classic proportions of the face as set out 2,500 years ago by the Greek geometer Pythagoras and refined in the 15th century by Leonardo da Vinci. We then will review the signs of aging and examine how different skin types age in differing ways and according to dissimilar timetables. We also will look at how society's perception of what constitutes beauty has changed in recent decades, with emphasis on what is most current today. Related facial plastic surgery procedures accompany illustrations, photographs, and charts.

If your analysis prompts you to read further, turn to part II for help in assessing your motivations for surgery and all-important information on how to choose a surgeon.

''As a layman, you need to have detailed information in order to sort out your role in the patient/doctor relationship,'' says the facial plastic surgeon from Michigan, cautioning that this role is different in self-elected surgery. ''This is not a medical emergency that dictates that you allow a more knowledgeable person—the surgeon—to decide whether surgery is indicated. You have time to study up on the situation.'' What you might expect of a first consultation also is covered in part II.

In part III, we will continue our examination of facial plastic surgery by discussing the most common surgical procedures. The benefits, risks, costs, and reactions of patients who have undergone these procedures will be carefully detailed.

What will people think if you elect to have surgery? You'll have to read part IV to find out.

I

Outer Image, Inner Beauty

1

The Proportions of Classic Beauty

CLASSIC BEAUTY. Adonis. Venus. Cleopatra. Catherine Deneuve. Brooke Shields. Robert Redford. Linda Evans.

These are the faces we all wish we had been born with, faces that undeniably earn a "10" in the rating scale vernacular of the twentieth century. But what is it about these faces that inspires our awe and our envy? Why are they "10s"?

"Beauty," says a California facial plastic surgeon, "is often said to be only skin deep. But I am here to tell you that true beauty goes clear to the bone."

That is because when talking about beauty, be it feminine beauty or masculine handsomeness, what really is being discussed is the underlying skeletal structure. It is the various dimensions of proportions and angles and contours and curves that work in harmony to create the concept of beauty.

A beautiful face is not determined by the skin, despite the time and energy we devote to skin care. It is what is under the skin, the skeletal

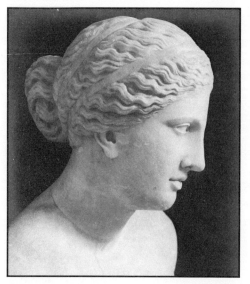 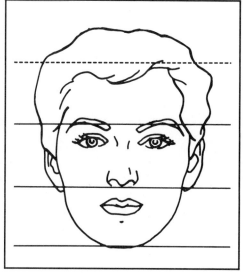

The Greek figure of Venus de Milo (c200 BC)   *Figure 1*
embodies the classic proportions of feminine
beauty.

structure, that makes the difference. Your facial plastic surgeon will spend a considerable amount of time analyzing your bone structure and facial features before discussing any possible improvements. That is why a surgeon might recommend a chin implant when the patient thinks he needs a rhinoplasty. In the end, the patient decides which procedures to have, but all patients should understand that the surgeon's advice is based on sound principles.

One such principle is that the perfect face can be divided into equal thirds. This is based on the mathematics of the golden proportion devised by the Greek mathematician Eudoxus and used since then in architecture and art. It was Pythagoras, another Greek mathematician, who determined that this formula also could be the basis for the portions of the human figure, and Leonardo da Vinci, some 2,000 years later, used this golden proportion to show that the face should be divided into three equal horizontal spaces. The famed artist showed how these spaces are further subdivided into spaces occupied by the facial features. Aesthetic balance is achieved when the facial features fall within these parameters (figure 1). To determine the "thirds," use a photograph and divide your face into three sections by drawing horizontal lines through the forehead hairline, the brow, the base of the nose, and at the lower margin of the chin. On the ideal face, the three sections are equal.

In determining the best look for a particular face, the facial plastic surgeon considers racial and ethnic differences. Although aesthetic principles may be said to hold true regardless of ethnic differences, the formulae for classic beauty are primarily relevant when applied to the Caucasian face. Just as the well-adjusted Caucasian woman does not want to look like an ingenue after surgery, neither does an Asian woman wish to take on a Nordic appearance or a black man the facial features of his white colleagues.

Because of his specialized training in the head and neck area, the facial plastic surgeon appreciates that ethnic sensibilities as well as differing customs and social norms are the foundation of aesthetic value. Bony structure is different for all races. Skin texture, color, and elasticity vary as well. A skilled surgeon acknowledges that racial qualities are appreciated differently in various cultures and makes no effort to impose racial limitations on beauty.

Nonetheless, balance and harmony in the face transcend ethnic and cultural differences, and an appreciation of what constitutes such balance among facial features is the first step in any surgeon's analysis of a patient's face.

Facial plastic surgeons also measure for full-face symmetry. While symmetry in the human face is rarely perfect, midline points should lie along a vertical line that splits the face. By dividing the face in halves and then fifths, the facial plastic surgeon can assess balance and symmetry (figures 2 and 3). The ideal face should be "five eyes wide," that is, five times the width of one eye. The space between the two eyes should be the width of one eye. In addition, the width of the nose should not extend beyond the lines drawn down from the inner corners of the eyes.

Evaluation of the five major masses—forehead, eyes, nose, lips, and chin—is considered essential in the aesthetic work-up prior to surgery.

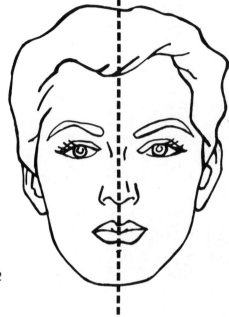

Figure 2

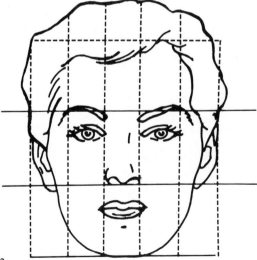

Figure 3

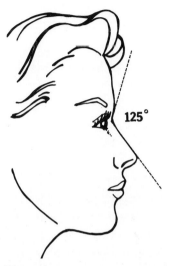

125°

Figure 4

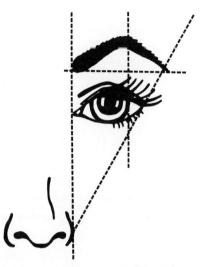

Figure 5

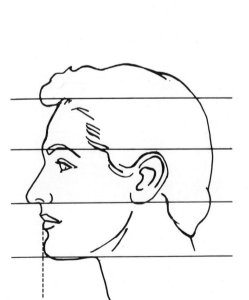

Figure 6

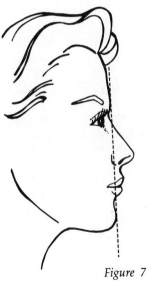

Figure 7

Among the factors to consider are the nasofrontal angle (figure 4), the brow in relation to the nose and the eyes (figure 5), the distances between the eyes and between the pupils of the eyes, the tip projection of the nose, and the length of the chin. To make your own chin evaluation, use a profile photo and draw a line straight down from your lower lip. For a man, the projection of the chin should be even with the lip (figure 6). For a woman, the chin should be slightly behind the line (figure 7).

Surgeons use a number of methods to evaluate a patient's face (figures 8 and 9), from complex mathematical calculations using profile and full-face photographs of the patient, to the use of instrumentation to assess the proper angles and projections.

The evaluation may vary according to the surgeon's own aesthetic sense. Not all plastic surgeons are artists, but the facial plastic surgeon possesses highly developed artistic sensibilities. Many take art courses and work in sculpture in preparation for a lifetime of redesigning and rejuvenating faces. They study faces, often subscribing to such magazines as Vogue and Glamour to keep up-to-date on current styles of beauty.

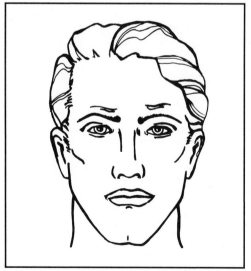

Figure 8

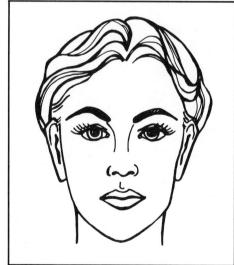

Figure 9

Styles Change; Style Doesn't

"What is beautiful changes constantly," one facial plastic surgeon notes. "It's fluid, it changes almost year to year—not changes just in how to dress a face but also what is considered a beautiful face structurally."

He notes, for example, that modeling agencies used to insist on the absolutely perfect, classic face. Today they prefer the occasional blemish or imperfection that lends character to a face. "Individuality is the key word for today's face. A natural look that maintains ethnic characteristics is preferred over 'carbon copy' looks adhering to Anglo-Saxon standards of beauty."

Finally, of course, are those men and women whose faces fail miserably in any test of classic beauty, yet they are spectacular to behold. That, say the facial plastic surgeons, is inner beauty. It simply cannot be reproduced.

2

The Signs of Aging

NEARLY EVERY WOMAN RECALLS VIVIDLY the first time she looked in a mirror and noticed a line at the corner of her mouth or near her eyes. No matter how self-assured or determined she was not to allow the external signs of beauty to control her life, she very likely felt a pang at the sight of that first wrinkle. Men often have the same reaction when they realize that their hairline is slowly receding or bags are developing under their eyes. Fine wrinkles around the corners of the mouth are one of the first signs of aging, and each decade brings more changes.

While the aging process itself cannot be changed, facial plastic surgery often can reverse some of its effects. The following charts delineate the signs of aging decade by decade and suggest appropriate corrective surgery.

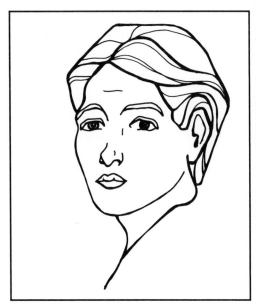

AGE 30

AGING SIGNS	CORRECTIVE SURGERY
EYES: Upper eyelids gradually become hooded. Pouching of lower eyelids becomes more prominent. Fine wrinkling begins	Eyelid surgery; collagen injections
FOREHEAD: Trace of frown lines in lower forehead and between eyes	Collagen injections; face sanding
MOUTH/LIPS: Fine wrinkling at outer corners	Collagen injections; face sanding; chemical peel
NOSE: Nose tip has not yet begun to droop with age, but shape of nose may suggest surgery	Nasal surgery

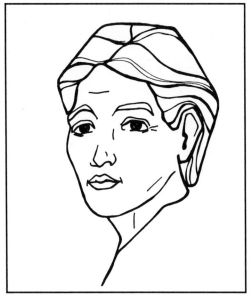

AGE 40

AGING SIGNS	CORRECTIVE SURGERY
EYES: Upper and lower eyelids begin to sag, creating deep-set look; crow's feet develop	Eyelid surgery
FOREHEAD: Frown lines deepen; horizontal wrinkles develop	Collagen injections; face sanding
MOUTH/LIPS: Vertical lines begin to appear and deepen around lips; wrinkling becomes more prominent	Chemical peel; collagen injections

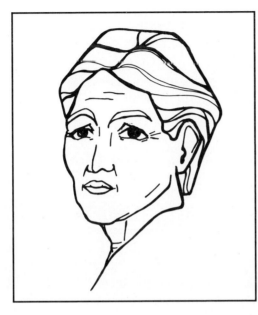

AGE 50

AGING SIGNS	CORRECTIVE SURGERY
CHEEKS: Fluid may accumulate in upper cheek area, causing pouches to form	Upper facelift; eyelid surgery
CHIN: Fat accumulates, creating a full, double chin	Chin surgery
EYES/EYEBROWS: Eyebrows sag, causing eyelids to appear hooded, heavy	Eyebrow lift; upper facelift
FOREHEAD: Horizontal lines now established; forehead sags	Forehead lift
JAWLINE: Jawline sags, creating the impression of jowls	Lower facelift
NOSE: Tip droops	Nasal surgery

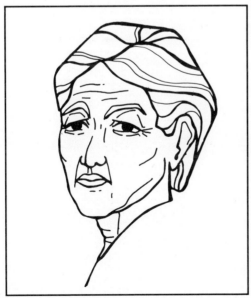

AGE 60+

AGING SIGNS	CORRECTIVE SURGERY
EYES: Eyelids sag further; hooded appearance becomes more pronounced	Eyelid surgery
FACE: Face loses elasticity; skin sags	Full facelift
FOREHEAD: Forehead lines deepen; temples deepen	Forehead lift
MOUTH/LIPS: Vertical wrinkling appears around lips	Chemical peel
NECK: Neck skin drops in folds; cords develop, creating a turkey-gobbler look	Lower facelift; neck lift

3

Effect of Skin Type on Facial Plastic Surgery

''DOCTOR, HOW WILL I LOOK WHEN MY SURGERY IS OVER?'' This is a common question, but not one easily answered since age, general health, skin quality, healing history, and degree of change sought all affect the final outcome. Ethnic background also affects the results of facial plastic surgery. Seven basic skin types have been identified, and all are affected in different ways by both the aging process and facial plastic surgery procedures. Asians, for example, show later signs of aging than Anglo-Saxons, but heal more slowly and sometimes develop thicker scars. It must be stressed that all facial plastic surgery in which incisions are required involves scarring. Often scarring is minimal, but it cannot be totally eliminated.

The following charts will help you evaluate how facial plastic surgery may affect you.

Guide to Skin Types

Here are the pros and cons of four of the most common facial plastic surgery procedures matched with skin type to help you decide if facial plastic surgery is for you.

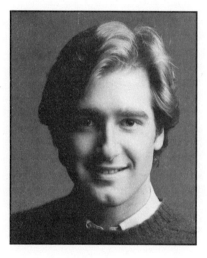

TYPE 1: Fair, dry, thin-skinned complexion (Anglo-Saxon)

FACIAL SURGERY (facelifts, scars, lesions)

PROS: Scars are usually quite thin. Skin drapes well for excellent facelift results.

CONS: Fine, deep wrinkling around mouth and eyes may be difficult to remove completely. Signs of aging appear early.

NASAL SURGERY

PROS: Thin skin allows more "chiseled" final result. Postoperative swelling and oiliness are minimal.

CONS: Any cartilage or bone irregularity is made more obvious.

EYEBROW LIFT

PROS: Heavy scars are rare.

CONS: Initial bruising is obvious. Fine "crepe" wrinkles may be a problem to remove.

DERMABRASION

PROS: Scars are always very thin, skin handles easily; slight pigmentation.

CONS: None.

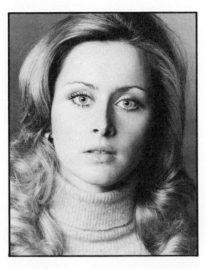

TYPE 2: Fair, blue-eyed, blond complexion (Northern European)
FACIAL SURGERY

PROS: Scars are thin, almost invisible. Skin heals well after facelift.

CONS: Fine, deep wrinkling may be difficult to completely remove around mouth and eyes. Signs of aging appear early.

NASAL SURGERY

PROS: Same as type 1.

CONS: Slightly thicker skin, but irregularities may still show.

EYEBROW LIFT

PROS: Any scars are very fine; heavy scars are very rare. Thin skin means easy surgical handling.

CONS: Initial bruising is obvious. Fine "crepe" wrinkles may be a problem to remove.

DERMABRASION

PROS: Same as type 1.

CONS: None.

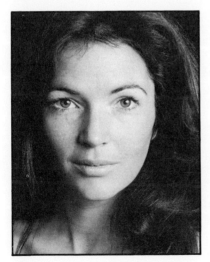

TYPE 3: Ruddy, freckled complexion (redhead)
FACIAL SURGERY

PROS: Fine scars usual. Signs of aging appear later.

CONS: Scar quality is somewhat less predictable; some chance of postoperative pigmentation.

NASAL SURGERY

PROS: Bone and cartilage structure usually is good.

CONS: More postoperative oiliness; may bruise easily; longer postoperative swelling.

EYEBROW LIFT

PROS: Fine scar lines are quite probable.

CONS: Heavier scarring may occur unpredictably. Fine, white scar may contrast with peach skin tone.

DERMABRASION

PROS: Any scars are fine and very thin.

CONS: Scars may appear heavier than in types 1 and 2. Some chance of postoperative pigmentation. Skin cancers are most common in this group.

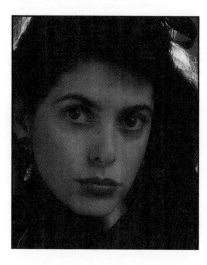

TYPE 4: Darker, oily, brunette complexion (Southern European)

FACIAL SURGERY

PROS: Fine scars are not unusual. Fine wrinkling over face is less common. Signs of aging appear later.

CONS: Scarring in front of and behind ears may be heavier. Heavier skin resists lifting somewhat. Darker scarring is more common.

NASAL SURGERY

PROS: Bone and cartilage structure are usually adequate.

CONS: Fine "chiseled" look not likely. Considerably longer postoperative swelling.

EYEBROW LIFT

PROS: Fine scars usually result. Fine wrinkling is less likely.

CONS: Scars may be thicker, bruising longer.

DERMABRASION

PROS: Skin cancers are less common.

CONS: Darker scarring is more common; heavier scarring is possible.

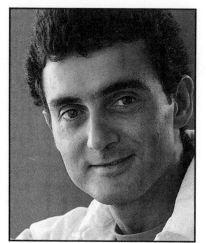

TYPE 5: Oily, olive, dark complexion (Greek, Turkish)

FACIAL SURGERY

PROS: Signs of aging appear later.

CONS: Heavy and darker scars are more common.

NASAL SURGERY

PROS: Bone and cartilage structure may be adequate.

CONS: Drooping cartilage structure resists change. Prolonged postoperative swelling and oiliness.

EYEBROW LIFT

PROS: Baggy eyelids may be less obvious.

CONS: Possible thicker scars. Bruise pigment may last.

DERMABRASION

PROS: Skin cancers are very rare.

CONS: Darker scarring is more common. Heavy or obvious scarring is more common.

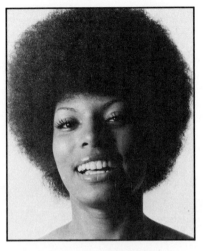

TYPE 6: Black complexion
FACIAL SURGERY

PROS: Signs of aging appear very late. No fine wrinkling.

CONS: Keloids (excessive tissue scarring) and dark or light pigmentation changes are possible. Heavy skin resists lifting.

NASAL SURGERY

PROS: Similar to type 5.

CONS: Cartilage structure prevents easy reconstruction.

EYEBROW LIFT

PROS: Baggy lids are less common.

CONS: Possible keloid formation.

DERMABRASION

PROS: Skin cancers are very rare.

CONS: Risk of keloids. Dark or light pigmentation changes are possible.

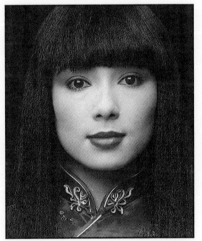

TYPE 7: Far Eastern complexion
FACIAL SURGERY

PROS: Signs of aging appear late. No fine wrinkling.

CONS: Same as type 4.

NASAL SURGERY

PROS: Similar to type 4.

CONS: Low nasal bridge problem.

EYEBROW LIFT

PROS: Symmetry and permanence of new eyelid creases through surgery.

CONS: Additional surgical steps are needed for creation of eyelid crease.

DERMABRASION

PROS: Similar to type 4.

CONS: Similar to type 4.

4

The Face of Today

WHEN SHANA C. FIRST MET with her facial plastic surgeon to discuss a narrower nose and more definitive cheekbones, she was adamant on one point. "I want to look like me when it's all over," she said, "not some caricature of Sandra Dee."

Shana—and thousands of other facial plastic surgery patients—have been pleased to find out that facial plastic surgery today results in a far more natural, less stereotyped appearance that capitalizes on the individual's own beauty, not some current film star's.

The ski-jump nose and slightly startled expression that typified the faces of many models who graced magazine covers in the 1950s and '60s have given way to a more natural, less artificial, and certainly more personalized look.

Fuller, richer lips, high cheekbones, and stronger chins are features the modern beauty strives for—whether achieved by great genes or enhanced through facial surgical techniques.

The face of today also might feature:
- narrower eyelids, probably including a ''more athletic'' upper eyelid;
- a stronger nose with a broader tip;
- a strong chin;
- more firmly defined cheekbones;
- hairlines that appear fuller and more natural;
- smaller earlobes; and
- better harmony and balance between the features and regions of the face.

''The concept of facial beauty has changed dramatically over the past 30 years from the childlike, dreamy look of the 1950s to today's natural, assertive individual look,'' comments a facial plastic surgeon from Birmingham, Ala. ''Established facial plastic surgery techniques are being refined constantly to achieve this 'nonsurgical' look, and new—in some cases revolutionary—techniques such as bone sculpting can achieve impressive results unheard of in past decades.''

Facial sculpting, the alteration of the underlying skeletal structure, is one of the newest and most exciting techniques available to today's patient. In the 1950s, facelifts could produce only surface skin tightening. Today, with the surgeon's ability to rework the muscles underlying the skin, remove offending fat, sculpt the bones, or insert implants to enhance the cheekbones or the chin, dramatic results are possible. Today, facial plastic surgeons can obtain 20 to 25 percent better results in facelifting than were possible 10 years ago.

Who are the candidates for these new procedures? Anyone who desires the latest look. Says a New York facial plastic surgeon, the change from the round-eyed look of the past to an ''intelligent, assertive, athletic eyelid . . . is the look of someone who is on the floor of the Stock Exchange. It is a normal look, the look of someone who works in the world.''

Most people who seek facial plastic surgery today are "very happy, well-adjusted, normal people who just want to look a little better," comments another facial plastic surgeon, from Beverly Hills, Calif. When they walk into his office, he says, these patients are more likely to say something like, "I don't want to look younger; I just want to look better."

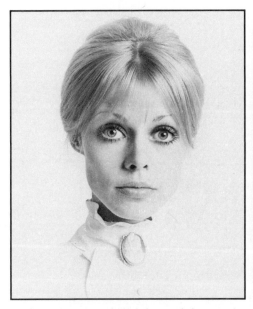 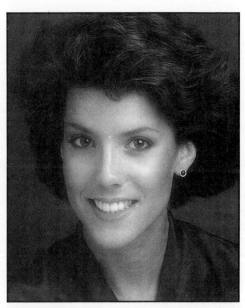

A ski-jump nose and slightly startled expression characterized beauty in the 1960s.

In the 1980s, a more natural, less artificial, and more individual look is desirable.

Facial Plastic Surgery and Beauty: an Evolution

	1950s and '60s	1970s	Today
EYEBROW/EYELID SURGERY	• high-lidded eyes • lots of space between eye and brow • wide-eyed look • incision line at corner of eye covered by "doe-eye" makeup • incision line visible • eyebrows raised very high	• lid width narrows, brow still slightly high • entire eyelid sculpted rather than lifted for more natural look	• narrower lid • 5 to 6 millimeters of space between brow for eye • natural appearance • incision line extends from upper lid, instead of corner of eye
FACELIFT	• surface changes only • pulled-back, stretched appearance • incision line visible	• underlying musculature tightened • incisions reconsidered for less obvious scarring • neckline scars still visible	• very natural, non-surgical look • complete scar camo-flaging • adjustments more sophisticated
FACIAL SCULPTING	• did not exist	• did not exist	• bone reshaped to improve facelift results • solves facial balance problems not addressed before
NOSE SURGERY	• turned up, ski-jump angle, nostrils showing • cute, childlike • highly sculpted tip	• transition from styl-ized, uniform result to more aggressive nose	• longer, stronger nose • 90% upward angle • wider bridge • fuller, gently refined tip • individualized nose based on each face • natural, non-surgical look

II

Is Facial Plastic Surgery for You?

5

Realistic Expectations

After watching women pass through a facial plastic surgeon's office as if negotiating a revolving door—walking in tiredly with wrinkles, bumps, and sags; marching out several weeks later with aplomb, rejuvenated, refreshed—a member of the office staff asked the surgeon, "If I get my weight down and have some facial plastic surgery, do you think I could be perfect?"

"Perhaps," he sagely replied, "but I'm not sure you want to be."

LOOKING GOOD—NOT PERFECT—is the goal of facial plastic surgery, and anyone who expects more is not a good candidate for surgery. Before you consult a surgeon, it is therefore wise to assess your own motivations. They are among the first topics your surgeon will discuss. Psychologists once believed that facial plastic surgery signaled a neurotic or even psychotic personality. Today they discount that theory for most patients, saying instead that cosmetic changes generally seem to have a healthful effect on self-esteem and self-confidence.

In part this is because the typical patient of past decades—older women who had just experienced grief; insecure men; and men and women who feared losing their jobs—has given way to a younger clien-

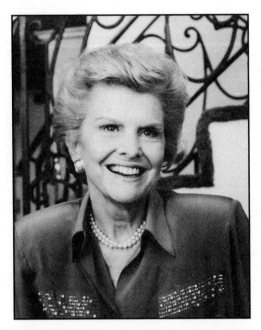

Former First Lady Betty Ford, in a long, personal assessment that included admission of an alcohol and drug dependency problem, decided that facial plastic surgery would give her a lift. She had the surgery for all of the right reasons and has proudly publicized the results ever since.

tele who tend to be more self-assured initially and far more realistic in their expectations of the surgery. In short, fewer people are seeking outright perfection. *Most just want to look better.* This is a healthy progression, psychologists report.

Nonetheless, as a patient, you may be asked to complete a detailed evaluation form which includes a psychological assessment followed by one or more interviews with the surgeon. The questions asked may seem irrelevant to you, possibly even impertinent. The purpose of the questionnaire, however, is clear. Surgeons need to weed out those patients who expect more than the surgery can deliver; they also are trying to identify patients who go from surgeon to surgeon seeking multiple operations and patients whose motivations are faulty (perhaps they are at the surgeon's office at the urging of a boyfriend or parent rather than because of personal conviction). Patients seeking to change obvious ethnic features also are questioned carefully. These are the people who are not likely to be good candidates for surgery, the ones who in all probability would

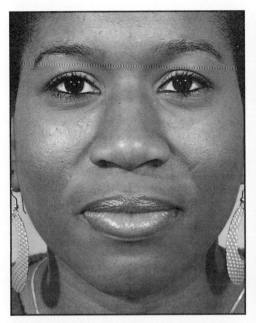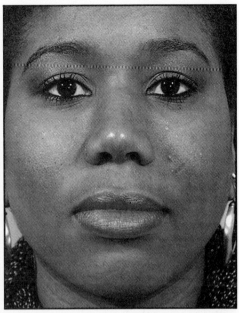

In a black patient, the surgeon should not try to obtain a Caucasian nose, but rather a more refined sculptured black nose.

not like the surgical results and may even feel guilty or angry at having gone through with it.

A made-for-television movie aired in early 1988, ''Perfect People,'' documented a married couple's decision to revamp their bodies and faces via exercise, plastic surgery, and diet. At one point the husband lamented, ''If we liked each other better, we wouldn't have to do all this.'' Actually, he missed the point. It is the individuals who do like themselves, who feel comfortable with who they are and what they have become, who are the best candidates for facial plastic surgery. They will not look to the surgery to cure insecurity and a low self-esteem.

The Psychology of Facial Plastic Surgery

Self-image is formed throughout life by a complex series of developmental and social experiences. Depending on one's early experiences with family and parents, his reaction to his appearance may be good or bad, pleasing or repulsive, liked or disliked. Society simply enforces this by placing great importance on external appearance. The slovenly appearing individual is deemed to be of lesser intelligence. The 50-ish woman in sturdy shoes and a no-nonsense hairdo is going to find the workplace a difficult nut to crack regardless of her skills and abilities. A man whose forehead furrows give him a perpetual scowl is believed to have a nasty disposition as well. Bags under the eyes often signal fatigue.

A famous sociologist and student of facial plastic surgery, Frances Cooke Macgregor, once observed that "so closely is the face tied to the core of the self . . . that any visual damage to it, minimal or severe, is normally accompanied by the pervading sense of shame and loss." Thus facial plastic surgeons must carefully assess if the prospective patient can emotionally withstand changes to the face.

Surgeons also must be attuned to the manner in which different cultures value different facial features. Macgregor tells the story of a young man of Spanish descent who sought reconstructive surgery for facial scars incurred in a motorboat accident. The surgeon attended to the forehead scarring in the first operation and then turned to the damaged nose. The patient, however, insisted that some rather minor scarring of the eyelids receive primary attention: "What bothers me most," he said, "is the sagging of my eyelids. It seems as though my eyes have lost their sparkle and life."

Self-evaluation

Facial plastic surgery should not be considered lightly simply because its purpose is to improve appearance; like any other surgery, it entails risks. This questionnaire will help you collect information about your physical condition, past medical history, habits, personality, etc., that will enable you to decide whether you should have surgery at the present time. The surgeon you choose may ask you to fill out a surgical evaluation form which may contain similar questions before agreeing to perform any facial plastic surgery on you.

1. What specific features do I want corrected?
2. How long have I been thinking about having surgery?
3. What caused me to begin thinking about it?
4. Is having surgery my idea or someone else's?
5. Why did I wait until now to consider the correction?
6. Do I understand that the object of any facial plastic surgery is to improve appearance, not to achieve perfection?
7. Do I feel embarrassed or guilty about having the operation?
8. Have I had any previous facial plastic surgery? Was I satisfied with the results?

Medical Evaluation

1. Have I ever experienced any unusual bleeding or poor scarring?
2. Have I suffered with recurrent nose bleeds?
3. Do I bruise easier than most people?
4. Has there been a recent emotional crisis in my life?
5. Am I on a special diet at the present time?
6. Have I ever had facial paralysis?
7. Do I have asthma or any chronic lung or bronchial conditions?

continued

Personality Inventory

1. Does life often seem burdensome to me?
2. Am I pessimistic about the future?
3. Do I often feel useless and unable to cope?
4. Do I often have fatigue or other physical symptoms that seem difficult to diagnose and relieve?
5. Do I have a tendency to let my imagination "run wild?"
6. Do I consider myself a person attuned to the dramatic aspects of life?
7. Do I consider myself an artistic or aesthetic person?
8. Have people said that I am unpredictable?
9. Have people said that I am an exciting person?
10. Do I spend a lot of time on my appearance?
11. Do I find myself stirring things up so that I become the center of attention?
12. Do I tend to deny my emotional needs?
13. Do I pride myself on being punctual? conscientious? self-critical? tidy? orderly?
14. Do I consider myself proud, strong, independent, and reserved; or dependent, warm, and affectionate?
15. Am I considered opinionated and stubborn?
17. Was I considered introverted as a teenager?
18. Do I try to help others and get hurt a lot?
19. Am I a social nonconformist, a "free spirit?"
20. Did I dislike school or consider it a waste of time?
21. Am I more comfortable when I understand why things happen?
22. Am I an opportunist?
23. Do I resist authority figures?
24. Deep down, do I consider myself to be endowed with superior, unique, or unrecognized abilities?
25. Was I considered a quiet, shy, obedient child?
26. Would I rather be alone than with people most of the time?
27. When discouraged, do I feel apathetic and indifferent?
28. Do I hold grudges?
29. Am I hypersensitive to the opinions of others?
30. Do I prefer to do things by myself rather than delegating them to others?

The surgeon considered the patient's demand for eyelid surgery first to be so bizarre, in light of the minimal damage to the eyelids, that he suggested the patient seek psychiatric help. However, what the surgeon did not take into consideration was the special significance that the eyes have for people of Spanish heritage. "In Spain," says Macgregor, "the eyes have special social significance. Described by Cervantes as 'silent tongues,' to the Spaniard they play a predominant role in communication, particularly in flirtations."

In the same vein, certain ethnic groups, such as those of Italian or Arabic heritage, place strong cultural identification on the nose. In fact, for males in general, the nose has certain sexual symbolism that may cause the patient extreme distress if altered surgically. It is significant that the three recorded murders and one attempted murder of plastic surgeons by their patients came at the hands of dissatisfied male rhinoplasty patients. Obviously, surgeons have reason to be cautious of patients with unrealistic desires.

But that does not mean that facial plastic surgeons reject all individuals with prominent ethnic features. Sometimes the operation can be a huge success, as was the case with Sam B.

Sam was a rather shy 39-year-old man born into an immigrant family, who felt that his oversized ethnic nose was detrimental in both business and social situations. He wanted a new identity that would not brand him as a foreigner. He wanted to fit into American society and escape the insulting jokes to which he was constantly subjected.

Sam's surgeon patiently explained that nasal surgery would not disguise his nationality; that was evident from his accented speech and many mannerisms. It was certainly possible for Sam to have a better looking nose, but no operation was going to change his personality.

"Well, Doctor," Sam said after pondering the surgeon's statements, "sometimes I don't feel so good about myself when I look into the mirror and see dark, unhappy, sad eyes peeking out from behind my mountain of a nose. I think my eyes could 'see' more if my nose was a hill rather than a mountain."

The doctor looked at Sam and had to agree that he had a beady-eyed appearance. He began to visualize what this man might look like if his nose was reduced to a rugged hill from an awesome Alp. No doubt people would respond to his appearance in a more positive manner if he no longer looked so intimidating. Sam proved to be a model patient, and by the time he returned for his "after" photograph a month after the surgery, he reported he had a new girlfriend and was hopeful it would develop into something special.

When a Surgeon Says, "No"

Of significance to the facial plastic surgeon is the patient's degree of self-esteem and commitment to having the surgery. When surgery is dictated by medical necessity, the patient often has little choice; at the very least, it is the physician who suggests that surgery is the best option. However, facial plastic surgery is elective surgery. It is the patient who requests the surgery and the physician who must ascertain if the surgery is important. Moreover, the surgeon must determine if the patient is attempting to solve psychological or other problems through external rather than internal means.

Nearly all surgeons are cautious about accepting several types of individuals as patients:

1. People with strange reasons for wanting the surgery.

A young man in his early 20s sought a facelift because his fellow assembly line workers made fun of him for being "too old," although his appearance was that of a normal, healthy 23-year-old. The surgeon refused to perform the operation, aware that he could not solve the young man's problem and, indeed, if his co-workers were to notice the scars of a facelift, they would tease him unmercifully.

2. Prospective patients who seem out of touch with reality.

An obese woman in her mid-30s was angry and surprised when a surgeon refused to perform eyelid surgery on her. The woman was bulging out of dirty jeans, wearing a stained blouse and filthy, worn sneakers. Her lusterless hair was dyed an unnatural color, and her makeup could only be described as overdone. She said she hated to look in the mirror and felt that if she had her eyelids done, she would be able to find a new boyfriend. The surgeon turned her down because, studying her, he could see a myriad of things she could do to improve her appearance, each one of which would do far more than surgery.

3. People who seek surgery at someone else's instigation.

Doctors' files are full of cases where a young girl, sullen and uncommunicative, is brought in by a beautiful mother who feels the daughter needs nasal surgery. Sometimes it is a wife whose husband has indicated she would look better after facial plastic surgery or even an employer who makes the suggestion. In such cases, doctors must probe deeply to discover whether the patient agrees.

4. People who have something in their mind's eye that the surgeon feels cannot be done.

One surgeon relates how he was on his way to the elevator in his office building when he was approached by a breathless old man who said he had just arrived on the bus from West Virginia and was desperate for a facelift and "whatever else was necessary." He acknowledged he did not have an appointment, but said he had heard of the surgeon from a relative who had had facial plastic surgery years before.

The man then proceeded to report that his wife had left him for a younger man, and his daughter had kicked him out of the house because he was too old. He was determined to do something about it and even was prepared to sell a piece of inherited property to pay the surgeon's fees. The surgeon felt sorry for this pathetic old man but refused to operate, since surgery obviously could not bring back what he most longed for: the love of his family.

Surgery is Forever

Why is it so important for the surgeon to assess prospective patients' motivations? Because, unlike an Elizabeth Arden makeover, the results of facial plastic surgery cannot simply be wiped off with cold cream and a tissue when the procedure is over. While implants can be readjusted or even removed, and second or even third surgeries are often necessary to refine a procedure, facial plastic surgery basically is a permanent solution. For personal, professional, and legal reasons, surgeons want happy—not dissatisfied—patients. Thus, they avoid performing surgery on individuals who are not likely to be happy with the surgical results.

Moreover, facial plastic surgery, unlike a cosmetic makeover, may involve a certain degree of discomfort and weeks—even months—of swollen tissues and bruising (the nose often does not lose all of its swelling and gain its final appearance for an entire year). New techniques have made it possible for most patients to resume normal activities in a short period of time, but no surgeon can totally predict how easily any one patient will heal. With certain procedures, such as hair flaps, the appearance may be worsened before it gets better.

No one walks into a facial plastic surgeon's office in the morning with baggy eyelids and a receding chin only to emerge that afternoon rejuvenated and born anew. The facial plastic surgery patient requires personal motivation, realistic expectations, and a certain degree of patience for the surgery to be considered truly successful. The patient and surgeon together must decide if facial plastic surgery is the correct solution.

6

Choosing a Facial Plastic Surgeon

"IT'S YOUR FACE. Why trust it to anyone but the best?" is the slogan of one popular advertisement for facial plastic surgery and, most would agree, it is eminently good advice. It is perfectly natural to want an outstanding facial plastic surgeon. The problem is finding one.

"I am amazed," says a facial plastic surgeon from Birmingham, Mich., "when the occasional patient still asks whether his or her choice of surgeon might truly affect the outcome of facial plastic surgery. Of course the surgeon makes a difference."

This is not to say that good results can be guaranteed by even the most highly qualified surgeon. Surgery is not an exact, predictable science, and results always will be affected by such factors as the patient's age, health, skin texture, bone structure, ability to heal, and the nature of the defect for which correction is sought. Good facial plastic surgeons are skilled at handling all of the unique conditions that each individual patient presents. The successful ones have reputations for superb results among former patients, medical colleagues, cosmeticians, and others, and it is to these people that you might first turn for a surgeon recommenda-tion. The names of surgeons also might become known to you through other sources, ranging from newspaper features to Yellow Pages listings.

Where to Find a Surgeon

To learn more about how people find facial plastic surgeons and what weight they give their sources of information, an independent survey recently was conducted by Market Facts, Inc., for the American Academy of Facial Plastic and Reconstructive Surgery. Here is a breakdown of how patients reported having found their surgeons:

1. Former patients, their families and friends

According to the Market Facts survey, only 40 percent of respon-dents considering facial plastic surgery said that they would rely on the recommendation of a friend or relative when choosing a surgeon. But one of the most valuable barometers of a surgeon's ability is his reputation among former patients, their families and friends. Good results speak loudly, and no surgeon can keep the doors open on an elective surgery practice unless he develops a large word-of-mouth referral network. Es-tablished facial plastic surgeons can document that 80 to 90 percent of their practice comes from patient referrals.

Getting a recommendation from a patient is not difficult. Bring up the topic of facial plastic surgery with enough people, and you will find someone who has had—or knows someone who has had—a facelift, nasal reconstruction, or some other procedure. You will be surprised at the amount of information volunteered about surgical procedures that people would not talk about only a few years ago.

It pays to track down several former patients. Most people will not regard an honest inquiry as an invasion of privacy, but it may be wise to ask the person who knows the former patient to call and ask if you can meet him or her to talk about the surgical experience. Most people who are willing to talk are genuinely interested in sharing both positive and negative surgical experiences, and you will glean valuable information from a few questions:

Art Versus Surgery

Must a facial plastic surgeon also be an artist? Can anyone learn facial proportions and planes, or is innate artistic talent a prerequisite for redesigning the face? Surgeons themselves don't agree, but two things are clear: An artistic sense is very helpful; a sensitivity to aesthetics and to current trends in beauty is essential.

One way you might gauge this is by paying close attention to office surroundings. The surgeon's office should have artistic decor that reflects a sense of harmony and good taste. Perhaps this was achieved at the hands of a decorator, but at least the surgeon realized its importance. Physicians who believe that a facial plastic surgeon is lost without a good eye for beauty and creative imagination might go a step further with fresh flower arrangements and special attention to music and the general ambiance.

A dignified, immaculately groomed staff reflects well on the physician's artistic nature; the physician himself should be impeccably attired and groomed. Selected pieces of quality artwork around the office may be the work of the surgeon himself.

How did you locate your surgeon?
Are you happy with the results?
Would you return to the same surgeon for another procedure?
What did the surgeon charge?
Were revisions necessary?
Keep a written list of comments about surgeons other people have consulted. It will help you when it is time for you to choose a facial plastic surgeon. If, during the course of your investigation, you begin to hear a long litany of complaints from many people about any single doctor,

rule that surgeon out right away. On the other hand, if you repeatedly see living proof of a surgeon's ability and like the results, that is a strong point in that surgeon's favor. Always keep in mind that you are seeking the superior surgeon who consistently gets good results. Continue to check around and narrow the field until you have located one or two highly recommended facial plastic surgeons, then interview them and select the surgeon whose "chemistry" seems to mix well with your own.

2. Medical referrals

Americans feel comfortable seeking referrals for specialized medical services from their "family doctors." Not surprisingly, in the same Market Facts survey, 86 percent of all respondents considering facial plastic surgery said they would ask another doctor to refer them to a facial plastic surgeon. About 40 percent said they would trust referrals from nurses or other medical personnel, and 27 percent named medical referral services as a good source.

The value of these sources is entirely dependent on the source's personal knowledge of the surgeon's skills and understanding of facial plastic surgery in general. Consistent good results still are the most important criteria.

Medical referral services may or may not provide complete details about a particular surgeon's qualifications, but they can provide a starting place—a list of all surgeons who are qualified under state law to perform the surgery you want. Reference sources include:

- *Directory of Medical Specialists,* possibly available at the local library.
- *County medical society referral service.* Callers usually are given the three names at the top of an alphabetized or regional list of surgeons who do this work. To assure all members an equitable number of referrals, the names at the top of the list then rotate to the bottom and three new names appear for the next caller. Therefore, this service will not provide a complete listing. Request the names of surgeons who limit their practice to the face.

- *National toll-free referral service.* By dialing a toll-free telephone number, United States or Canadian residents can receive a list of board-certified facial plastic surgeons who practice in their state or province, as well as a free brochure on any procedure they are considering. Staffed by the Facial Plastic Surgery Information Service, the referral service numbers are:

In the U.S.: (800) 332-FACE

In Canada: (800) 523-FACE

In the District of Columbia: 842-4500

Many medical practitioners have had firsthand opportunity to witness facial plastic surgery and can offer expert testimony as to how well and how often a surgeon performs the particular procedure you want. But be sure this personal knowledge backs any recommendation given you.

Facial plastic surgery is a relatively new facet of a highly specialized profession and, even among the general medical community, may not be well known. When that is the case, even doctors can make blind faith assumptions about other doctors, as this story from a Michigan facial plastic surgeon illustrates:

"A fellow doctor related to me how he sent his daughter to a good friend of his, a general plastic surgeon with a good reputation for hand surgery, for a consultation concerning a rhinoplasty. The girl elected to pursue surgery with her father's blessing. No one ever thought to ask this doctor friend how often he had performed nose correction surgery because they mistakenly thought that if a surgeon was good at one technique, he would be good at all others.

"The consequence was that too much cartilage was removed from the girl's nose, leaving her altered appearance in worse shape than her original nose. The doctor's second attempt to repair the damage resulted in additional problems, after which the father informed the general plastic surgeon, his former friend, that he would never send him another referral."

Some medical practitioners, like some people anywhere, look down on facial plastic surgery, especially cosmetic procedures. They do not have to live with the problem you are experiencing, and, unless they have known someone whose life changed for the better after successful facial plastic surgery, they may spend more energy trying to talk you out of surgery than finding you a qualified surgeon. Their recommendations should be taken with the proverbial grain of salt.

3. Yellow Pages or other advertisements

Would you choose your facial plastic surgeon from an advertisement, whether it was a listing in the telephone Yellow Pages or a professional medical newsletter mailed to your home? A relatively small number of individuals—6 percent according to the Market Facts survey—say they would seek a surgeon's name from the Yellow Pages or other advertisements, although 71 percent reported that they consider advertisements a good source of general information about facial plastic surgery.

Medical advertising has been permitted legally only since the late 1970s, and many consumers who remember when doctors did not advertise are not entirely comfortable with the idea. They may feel it smacks of hucksterism rather than merely being a way to introduce oneself to potential patients.

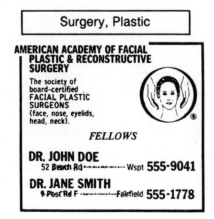

Physicians themselves are divided on whether advertising is an appropriate avenue for reaching patients. Some see in it a too facile way to bypass the long years of building a reputation through good results. As a facial plastic surgeon from Tacoma, Wash., says, "Prestige is not a commodity that can be purchased in the marketplace. It is something that must be earned through quality patient care over time."

Others see it as a necessary way to establish a practice in a new locale or simply to gain visibility in an overcrowded profession. In today's mobile society, many consumers find themselves without the personal contacts to locate a surgeon. Surgeons also sometimes turn to advertising when they have decided to change their specialty or their office location or have a new service to offer. Highly reputable facial plastic surgeons who advertise generally follow guidelines published by the American

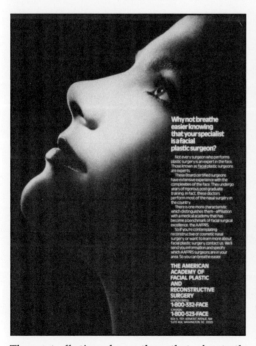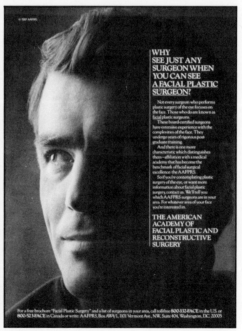

The most effective ads are those that educate the consumer.

Academy of Facial Plastic and Reconstructive Surgery—guidelines you also might follow when assessing the surgeon behind any advertisements you see:

- Advertisements should include only information that a reasonable person might regard as relevant to selecting a surgeon, such as physician specialty, board certification, description of services, range of fees for specific services, payment plans, and so on.
- Advertisements will exclude statements or photographs that promote relief unobtainable by the average patient, testimonials that do not reflect the typical experience of patients, and claims that take improper advantage of a person's fears, vanity, anxiety, or similar emotions.

You should be particularly skeptical of any advertisement that proclaims a surgeon or group of surgeons are the "only board-certified" plastic surgeons in a city. Such advertisements may be designed to deceive consumers into believing that only one specialty board certifies competence in facial plastic surgery. In reality, several such boards examine surgeons for competence in the field.

In most areas, surgeons who perform facial plastic surgery are listed in the Yellow Pages under one of two headings: "facial plastic surgeons" or "plastic surgeons." In some areas, facial plastic surgeons also are listed under "surgery—head and neck" and "otolaryngology." You might consider surgeons from any of those categories, but in narrowing down your list, keep in mind that you are looking for an experienced surgeon who mainly does facial plastic surgery and regularly performs the specific operation(s) you desire.

4. Hairdressers, cosmeticians, and manicurists

Although only 2 percent of respondents to the Market Facts survey said they would ask for a surgeon referral from someone in the beauty industry, the truth is that a good hairdresser may know a great deal about facial plastic surgery. During the course of their work, hairdressers see many facelift and eyebrow lift scars and often hear about the surgical experience over a shampoo and haircut. Since many women keep weekly hairstyling appointments, the hairdresser is actually able to witness the week-to-week healing process and can thereby render intelligent judgment of the overall results.

Cosmeticians and manicurists also come in contact with beauty-conscious women who willingly talk about their eyelid surgery, rhinoplasty, or collagen treatment. If you do not know anyone at all who has had the facial plastic surgery you wish to have, you might inquire at beauty shops around town to see who those ''in the know'' recommend.

Women who care about their appearance usually are willing to share some of their beauty secrets—such as their surgeon—with those truly interested in finding the best.

What Credentials Should I Look For?

There are plastic surgeons and there are facial plastic surgeons, and it is well worth the time to learn the difference, as this story from a Michigan facial plastic surgeon illustrates:

A family arranged to have the university chief of plastic surgery redo the son's nose. As a burn specialist, he had a formidable reputation, but as a facial plastic surgeon, he failed the task. After three tries, he still was unable to produce satisfactory results, and the parents were obliged to take the unfortunate son elsewhere for the necessary repair.

Facial plastic surgeons devote their medical training and practice to performing a particular set of procedures (plastic surgery) on a certain region of the anatomy (the face and neck). To see if a surgeon you are considering is such a specialist, look at his credentials.

"Patients should feel free to ask a surgeon about his credentials," says another facial plastic surgeon, who practices in Miami Beach, Fla. "Good facial plastic surgeons are pleased to have the opportunity to build rapport with prospective patients, and they understand that the best way to do that is by establishing their credentials."

Health consumers today usually are aware of the importance of seeking a physician who is certified in the specialty that encompasses their medical needs. However, not many are aware that many specialists in facial plastic surgery are actually certified in otolaryngology-head and neck surgery and, as such, are specialists of the complex head and neck region. In comparison, surgeons certified in general plastic surgery are trained to perform plastic surgery over the entire body and may or may not specialize in the region of the face at all, as the previous anecdote clearly illustrates.

In surgery, as in anything else, practice makes perfect. "If I wanted my face done," the surgeon from Michigan notes, "I'd much rather find a surgeon who does 200 nose reconstructions a year than one who does only 20, and so should anyone else."

Other Credentials to Look for:
- *F.A.C.S. designation*: Fellowship in the American College of Surgeons.
- *Medical school faculty position*: Some of the most pioneering surgeons in the development of facial plastic surgery have been affiliated with medical schools. Such a position, though, is no guarantee of surgical results.
- *A.A.A.H.C. designation*: Surgeons with their own office surgery facilities increasingly seek accreditation from outpatient-oriented organizations such as the Accreditation Association for Ambulatory Health Care, Inc.

"Just remember," cautions the facial plastic surgeon from Michigan, "a long list of accolades does not measure proficiency in the operating room. Results are what count."

7

The Initial Consultation

HELEN WAS IN HER MID-20s, the mother of a busy set of two-year-old twins who accompanied her when she came to the surgeon's office to inquire about a nose reduction. She felt she had been cursed with a large, hooked nose. "If only I had a normal-sized nose without the hump, I would be much more attractive," she stated firmly.

The surgeon studied her features and then her profile and gently inquired if she had ever considered building up her receding chin line to draw attention away from her nose. "Oh yes," she said. "My dentist has already referred me to an oral surgeon who will correct my overbite, and that will bring my entire jaw forward. But I think nasal surgery would be the frosting on the cake."

The surgeon agreed. Helen had beautiful blue eyes and a proportionate mouth and cheekbones. With a smaller, straighter nose she would indeed look better. The surgeon explained what she should expect in the way of results and scheduled the surgery for two weeks hence.

From the moment the cast was removed—despite the swelling—Helen was completely satisfied with the results. By the time of her six-month checkup, she had undergone oral surgery and appeared transformed.

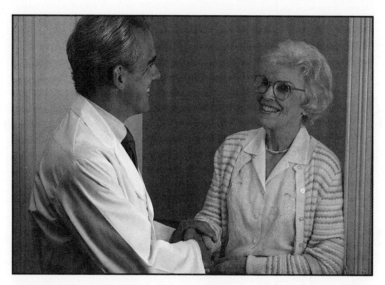

A comfortable relationship with each patient in pleasant—and private—surroundings is the atmosphere good surgeons strive for.

The ideal consultation is one that proceeds as Helen's did, with the patient able to articulate what he or she wants, the surgeon helpful and considerate with advice, and a harmony that develops between them.

Once you have narrowed your list to a possible surgeon, it is time to proceed with the consultation. If you have selected two surgeons as possibilities, suggests a facial plastic surgeon from Birmingham, Mich., save your top choice for last, so you will not need to make a return visit should you decide to schedule surgery. When you call ahead for an appointment, ask for brochures or pamphlets pertaining to the type of surgery that interests you. Most doctors will send these to you prior to your visit so you can prepare to ask questions about anything you find unclear. Read this literature carefully so you will be aware of the nature of the physician's practice.

If you have not already done so, now is the time to question the doctor or office staff about the doctor's background. If you are unfamiliar with his qualifications, you may ask for his curriculum vitae. This is his resume, which lists his education, training, teaching appointments, publications, and so on. It could be mailed to you along with any pre-consultation documents or information.

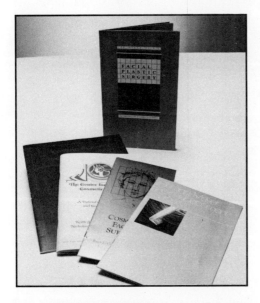

Facial plastic surgeons generally have a plethora of brochures available; many also have a brochure outlining specific office routines. Ask for these and read them carefully before your initial visit.

Consider having your spouse or a close friend accompany you on your initial consultation visit, but leave your young children with a sitter; the presence of fidgety youngsters is distracting both for you and the surgeon. A supportive friend not only can ease your mind while you wait to be seen, but also can remember details during the consultation itself that you may overlook in your nervousness. Good company will help you relax and, as a bonus, you will have another person's opinion of the surgeon. Your companion should be allowed into the consultation room with

Computerized Changes

Imagine being able to see your "after" photograph during the initial consultation, before surgery ever takes place. Through the wonders of space-age technology, a process known as computer imaging comes close to making that possible.

Using a computer, high-resolution monitor, video camera, special software, and an electronic sketch pad, the facial plastic surgeon can display the patient's image on the screen and then transform the facial features with the stroke of a lightpen or "mouse." Theoretically, the patient can "try out" several nose shapes or chin implants via the computer before the scalpel is ever taken in hand.

Surgeons who use this equipment claim it works well as long as the patient is aware of its limitations; that is, the computer can superimpose an image, but the software is not yet sophisticated enough to take into account underlying bone and muscle structures. Moreover, the computer cannot replicate a patient's healing capacity. Many surgeons are skeptical, however, noting that the computerized image may give patients false expectations. They claim that a simple artist's sketch of the proposed surgery is as valid and useful as the changes projected by computer imaging.

Despite the controversy, more and more surgeons are acquiring the equipment, so you, too, may get a chance to glimpse tomorrow today.

you, with the freedom to ask questions. But do not let your friend or family member monopolize the conversation. The surgeon needs to hear what you want done, not what someone else thinks you want done. This often is a problem when a mother or both parents accompany a teenager.

This was the case when Elizabeth, who appeared unhappy and withdrawn, arrived with her parents for a consultation at a busy surgeon's office. Her mother went on and on about how her daughter needed her nose fixed so she could lead a normal life, so she would accept herself, and so on.

Turning his back on her folks, the surgeon asked Elizabeth, "What can I do for you?" In a very small voice, the girl replied, "I wish I had another nose. All the kids at school call me hose nose, the anteater, or Betty Beak. Can you make my nose smaller?"

The surgeon assured her that he could, but that there was no guarantee it would be the nose of her dreams. "Doctor, anything would be better than what I have now," she wailed. The operation turned out to be a success, and Elizabeth was overjoyed at the sight of her new nose: It was love at first sight.

During the consultation, pay attention to the physician's staff, who should be both friendly and efficient. You may have more contact with these assistants than the doctor himself, since specific duties such as suture and nose cast removal often are delegated to a scrub nurse or medical assistant. Staff members also handle most of the routine consultation procedures; sometimes an assistant will take your medical history as well. Other duties of the office staff may be to take "before and after" photographs, show you the surgeon's collection of prior patient photos, make appointments, schedule surgery, and explain insurance forms.

The Consultation Begins

The consultation with the doctor allows you to evaluate the doctor's personality, age, manner, and methods. During this interview, you should feel comfortable with him, and he should exhibit an interest in you. You want a caring and considerate physician who answers all of your questions in nonmedical terms, who seems competent and organized, and who takes the time to be complete.

The facial plastic surgeon from Michigan recommends making an appointment with at least two surgeons so you can compare how each treats you during the initial visit. It will cost more money to visit two surgeons

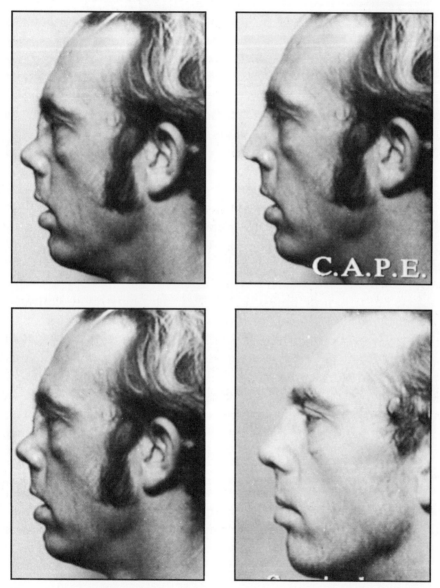

Computer imaging can help the patient visualize what the surgery may accomplish: Above, patient before surgery and as pictured after surgery by computer imaging; below, patient before and after surgery. Note that the surgeon's results are better than the computer's.

but will enhance your assurance that you have selected the most suitable surgeon for your individual needs.

Some doctors have impeccable credentials on paper but are brusque and arrogant in person. You should select a surgeon with whom you feel compatible, one who seems responsive to your wishes. If you are comfortable with neither physician, keep looking! Your face is too important for a second-rate decision.

The better surgeons tend to have perfectionist personalities, and this is to your benefit since they, too, want excellent results. Since they are more conservative and exacting by nature, they are usually more reserved in manner and dress. It is this very patience and frankness that give many patients a feeling of confidence in them. Doctors who are well-known, flamboyant playboys and nightowls cause considerable worry to patients who wonder what shape the surgeon will be in on the morning of their surgery.

Some highly competent surgeons continue operating well into their 70s, but if you feel uncomfortable about a surgeon's age, it may be better to cross him off your list. On the other hand, some patients do not want a young doctor fresh out of medical school either. In the final analysis, much depends on the personal chemistry that develops between the patient and the surgeon.

Another way to judge the surgeon is to focus on how he handles patients—his bedside manner. It is important that he takes ample time with you and encourages you to ask questions. Many people are in awe of doctors and are afraid to speak up. A good physician will sense this and will begin explaining the appropriate procedure, possible complications, fees, aesthetics, and so on, until a question pops into your head. You should feel enough at ease to question anything that you do not understand. You should not feel rushed.

A Picture Is Worth a Thousand Words

You may have an opportunity during the consultation to view ''before and after'' photographs of the doctor's representative surgical examples. As you study the photos, consider the face and features with which the physician had to work—the ''before'' photo. A good surgeon should be able to improve a person's looks to a certain degree. However, if a person is ugly to begin with, it is unreasonable to assume that any surgeon—even a top-notch one—will be able to transform such a person into someone of great classic beauty.

As you examine the comparison photos, try to disregard the difference in hairstyles and makeup (cover them with your hand if possible). So many patients feel better about their new look that they go out almost immediately and make additional changes, such as in hair coloring, styling, or makeup.

Because hairstyle and makeup may influence your judgment concerning the success of the surgery, you will have to make a conscious effort to focus on the line and form of the surgical change. All of the photos should show the person with the same lighting and at the same angle so you have an honest measure of the facial improvement accomplished.

If the nose has been corrected, check to see if it looks ''surgical,'' that is, too scooped out, too turned up with nostrils showing, too pinched at the tips, or nostrils pulled up on the side. If you are examining the results of eyelid surgery, check to see that the bottom eyelid does not show too much eye white. For facelifts, note if the skin appears drawn, creating an artificial appearance. Since skin and tissues stretch to accommodate the normal functions of chewing and smiling, the initial unveiling of a facelift may appear somewhat tight. Several months later, when the ''after'' photo customarily is taken, facial expression should appear entirely natural.

If you agree that the ''after'' photos of the surgeon's patients show a satisfactory degree of improvement, you most likely will be satisfied with the amount of your own surgical change. If you honestly think the photos do not show the kind of results you want, by all means go elsewhere.

What if the surgeon will not show you ''before and after'' photos of other patients? Chances are he does not have releases from his patients to show their pictures, and he is respecting their right to privacy. If photos are shown, you can be assured that patients have signed releases permitting the surgeon to use those photos to educate patients such as yourself.

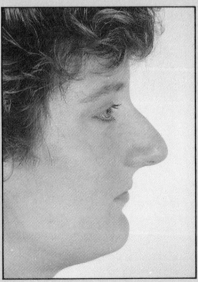 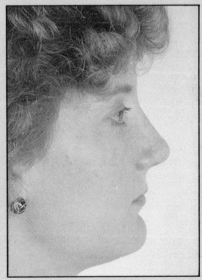

Before and after photos can help you evaluate the surgeon's skill.

The Risks of Surgery

Any surgical procedure involves some risk, such as bleeding, infection, or reaction to anesthesia, and your facial plastic surgeon should discuss these to your satisfaction.

However, patients should keep in mind that surgery is a two-way street. Just as the surgeon has a responsibility to tell you what possible risks the surgery entails, so have you a responsibility to level with the surgeon about your own health problems, such as bleeding disorders, heart disease, and diabetes, and personal habits such as smoking, drinking, and heavy use of aspirin. If you don't tell your surgeon about all of your illnesses and medication that you take regularly, you may experience complications or poor results that could have been avoided.

For example, Shirley T. was scheduled for a facelift, rhinoplasty, and eyelid surgery—all at once. The hospital performed the usual screening tests, and the results were all in order. During the operation, the surgeon realized as soon as the blood pooled up at the first incision that something was wrong. It was necessary to re-open the facelift to close off the bleeders. Luckily, Shirley did not require a transfusion (she later admitted she had bled for a week after a tooth was pulled), but it is scary to think what might have happened had she hidden her medical history as a bleeder from a less-experienced surgeon.

Omitting facts about health problems could endanger your life.

The Issue of Privacy

A facial plastic surgeon from Tacoma, Wash., notes that patients should feel as if they are being treated with respect, consideration, and dignity. An important facet is the right to privacy, especially important since facial plastic surgery patients are working to improve self-image and self-confidence, which are very personal concerns.

"I tell my staff that I want them to be two things to a patient," he notes, "a hostess and a travel agent, because they [the patients] are taking a little trip toward self-improvement, and how it is arranged will certainly contribute to their degree of satisfaction." Privacy, he holds, includes the right to enter and leave the doctor's office unnoticed, to a private consultation room where the patient's true feelings can be expressed, to a private locker where personal things can be safely stowed away during the operation, and to a private recovery room—not one filled with the relatives of two or three other recovering patients.

Patients who value their privacy might prefer to have the surgery in an office or ambulatory facility rather than a hospital. The hospital, after all, is an on-stage performance with all sorts of operating room personnel, the admission and discharge procedure, and recovery rooms that may hold 10 to 15 people. This can be very depersonalizing in contrast to the private, caring atmosphere that often exists in an office facility.

The average consultation lasts between 20 minutes and a half hour. One visit may be sufficient, but either the doctor or patient may feel a second visit would be beneficial. Some doctors routinely schedule two visits about two weeks apart to go over all the details and to reassure the patient. The cost of the average consultation varies with the reputation of the surgeon and the part of the country where he practices (surgeons on the coasts tend to charge higher fees). An average fee would range between $50 and $100 and may or may not be deductible from the overall cost when surgery is scheduled. If you are concerned about the consultation fee, be sure to ask about it when you call for your initial appointment.

While you are engrossed in evaluating the doctor, he will be studying you as a prospective patient. Not everyone is a good candidate for

Patient Bill of Rights

(Reprinted here is a sample patient bill of rights courtesy of a facial plastic surgeon from Beverly Hills, Calif., which was written in accordance with California statutes.)

The patient can expect to:

1. Exercise these rights without regard to sex or cultural, economic, educational, or religious background or the source of payment for his care.
2. Receive considerate and respectful care.
3. Have knowledge of the name of the physician who has primary responsibility for coordinating his care and the names and professional relationships of other physicians who will see him.
4. Receive information from his physician about his illness, his course of treatment, and his prospects for recovery in terms he can understand.
5. Receive as much information about proposed treatment or procedure as he may need in order to give informed consent or to refuse this course of treatment. Except in emergencies, this information should include a description of the procedure or treatment, the medically significant risks involved in the treatment, alternate course of treatment or nontreatment and the risks involved in each, and the name of the person who will carry out the procedure or treatment.
6. Participate actively in decisions regarding his medical care. To the extent permitted by law, this includes the right to refuse treatment.

7. Full consideration of privacy concerning his medical care program. Case discussion, consultation, examination, and treatment are confidential and should be conducted discreetly. The patient has the right to be advised as to the reason for the presence of any individual.

8. Confidential treatment of all communications and records pertaining to his care and his stay in the hospital. His written permission shall be obtained before his medical records can be made available to anyone not directly concerned with his care.

9. Receive reasonable responses to any reasonable requests he may make for service.

10. Be allowed to leave the hospital even against the advice of his physicians.

11. Have reasonable continuity of care and to know in advance the time and location of appointment as well as the physician providing the care.

12. Be advised if hospital/personal physician proposes to engage in or perform human experimentation affecting his care or treatment. The patient has the right to refuse to participate in such research projects.

13. Be informed by his physician or a delegate of his physician of his continuing health care requirements following his discharge from the hospital.

14. Examine and receive an explanation of his bill regardless of source of payment.

15. Know which hospital rules and policies apply to his conduct as a patient.

16. Have all patient's rights apply to the person who may have legal responsibility to make decisions regarding medical care on behalf of the patient.

facial plastic surgery (see chapter 5). Every year a facial plastic surgeon sees hundreds of prospective patients who display a tremendous diversity of reactions and behavioral patterns. In reaching a decision about whether the patient will be a good candidate for surgery, the surgeon must function somewhat as a psychologist. Over time and with experience, he becomes adept at assessing when any given patient's behavior is apart from the norm. If a surgeon says ''No'' to your request for facial plastic surgery, do not consider it a personal rejection; it is merely serious advice to reconsider the risks versus the goals you hope to attain.

Stating the Obvious

At the start of the consultation, when the doctor asks, ''What can I do for you?'' it is wise to give a straightforward answer. Tell him exactly what you hope to have done. The more you beat around the bush, rambling on about why you hate your sagging face or long nose, the more he will begin to worry about your motivation and expectations. It is sufficient to state that you feel your face would look better if you had the desired facial plastic surgery done.

If you have brought along any photos of your ''ideal'' nose or whatever, pull them out now for discussion. Although many doctors dislike patients bringing photos, claiming this shows a tendency toward unrealistic expectations, others believe that such photographs are useful if they help the patient show the doctor what they have in mind. Photographs are acceptable as long as the patient realizes that each surgery is a customized job to fit the individual; surgeons cannot put a movie star's nose on someone else's face.

A major purpose of the consultation, of course, is to have the surgeon examine the condition you wish to have changed. Only then can he tell you what he believes can be accomplished by surgery in your particular situation. Since this is a highly individual analysis, factors such as your age, health, skin texture, bone structure, and healing capacity all must be taken into account.

Practice Makes Perfect

If at the end of the consultation you feel you are on the same wavelength as the surgeon, ask the consultation clincher: How often does he perform the type of facial plastic surgery you wish to have?

A surgeon of the best quality should perform at least 50 nose corrections a year and a minimum of 25 facelifts and 50 eyelid surgeries. Of course, quantity cannot be equated with quality. Some surgeons handle fewer cases than average and charge more to make up the difference in income. The best advice is to avoid surgeons who turn out patients on an assembly line basis as well as those who perform the procedures infrequently.

Different surgeons use different methods of examination and explanation. Some use protractors to measure the nose; some project photos on a screen; some make elaborate masks and casts. Don't be overly impressed with gimmicks that measure or mold your features. According to the surgeon from Michigan, a competent surgeon doesn't need these for visualization purposes; they are most often used to allay the concerns of the patient. A simple sketch probably is all a surgeon needs in conjunction with your "before" medical photo. He may actually take this into the operating room with him to use as a reference.

As the patient, you will be provided detailed information concerning the diagnosis and likely outcome of the surgical procedure. Facial plastic surgery patients, says the surgeon from Washington, are often more educated, more interested in the technical details of the surgery. Questions run the gamut of how much pain is involved to what type of anesthesia, how soon will the patient look presentable, and what possible complications could result.

Paying the Bill

Surgeons vary widely in the fees they charge for facial plastic surgery procedures, with the highest fees likely to be charged on either coast and by surgeons who have acquired a reputation for quality work.

The actual cost will depend on a number of factors, including the extent and complexity of the surgery, the skill and experience of the surgeon, where the surgery is performed (fees tend to be highest in New York, California, and Florida), the type of anesthesia used, and whether a hospital stay is involved.

Under the law, surgeons set their own fees; no organization sets fees for facial plastic surgery. Your facial plastic surgeon or his staff will inform you of costs at your initial consultation. However, as a generalized guide, here are some price ranges exclusive of hospital, anesthesia, nursing care, and medication:

4 eyelids (upper and lower)	$2,000—$4,000
2 eyelids (upper or lower)	$1,000—$4,000
Facelift (not including eyelids)	$2,000—$10,000
Eyebrow-lift	$1,000—$2,000
Chin implant	$ 500—$2,000
Neckline liposuction	$ 500—$1,500
Nose	$1,500—$6,000
Ears (both)	$1,000—$4,500
Cheek implants	$1,500—$2,500
Chemical peel (full face)	$1,000—$4,500
Dermabrasion (full face)	$1,000—$3,500
Collagen injections	$ 200—$ 350 (per visit)
Hair transplants	$ 15—$ 50 (per plug)
Scalp reduction	$ 600—$2,000

"We are sometimes asked about the consequences of not having surgery," he says. "I always say, 'Well, you can have facial plastic surgery to improve or maintain a good appearance, or you can simply accept the natural wrinkling that comes with aging.' "

Available services and office procedures will also be explained to you, including provisions for after-hour and emergency care and how to express grievances if you are dissatisfied with the surgery. Fees may be discussed by the surgeon or later by a member of the office staff.

It is extremely important that you, the patient, understand that most purely cosmetic procedures are not covered by medical insurance policies; moreover, facial plastic surgeons normally request payment in advance of the surgery. Some problems, such as a nasal deformity resulting from injury, birth defect, or hooded eyelids that interfere with vision, may be partially or even completely covered by insurance. But since a multitude of insurance policies exists, you must know the limits of your coverage and any restrictions, including requirements for second opinions.

The facial plastic surgeon from Washington recalls a patient who was having nasal surgery that should have been covered partially by her insurance. The insurance company would not pay, however, because the patient had not satisfied the waiting period on her policy. There is no way that the surgeon or his staff can be aware of these problems; patients should discuss the proposed surgery in detail with their insurance representatives before undergoing any surgery.

After your consultation is completed, you will be taken to the photography room where one of the staff members will take the "before" photo for your medical file. It is best to keep your face in natural repose—not grimacing, smiling broadly, or winking—so the surgeon will be able to see and study every wrinkle, line, and sag that is normally present without exaggerated facial expression.

If you decide to proceed with the surgery, you will be asked to sign certain legal forms. An informed surgical consent form is necessary for legal purposes. It gives the surgeon permission to perform the surgery and states that you have been informed about the procedure, possible complications, and alternative methods of treatment. Before signing, be sure you have a full understanding of the procedure contemplated. Some states allow medical arbitration as a legal alternative to the traditional judge and jury system. If you live in such a state, you will be asked to sign this form. You also may be asked to sign a form allowing the surgeon to show your photographs to others.

Once the initial consultation is over and you have made your decision, mull it over if you wish with your spouse or a close friend, preferably the one who accompanied you. But keep in mind that the final decision must be yours. It is your face that will undergo the operation.

Sample Informed Surgical Consent Form for Facial Plastic Surgery

NAME: _____

DATE:_____ TIME:_____ A.M._____ P.M._____

1. I hereby request and authorize Dr._____aided by any assistants that he may require to perform in the presence of qualified medical personnel to perform facial plastic surgery on me, on or about the___day of, _____19___, for the purpose of attempting to improve my facial appearance with respect to the following condition:_____
for which the following surgery will be performed:

_____

2. Dr. _____ has fully explained in terms clear to me the effect and nature of the operation to be performed, and foreseeable risks involved, and alternative methods of treatment. Lastly, I have been given an opportunity to ask any questions I desired regarding the matters covered in the preceding two sentences, and these questions have been answered to my satisfaction.

3. I also authorize the operating surgeon to perform any other procedures which he may deem necessary or desirable in attempting to improve the condition stated in paragraph one or any unhealthy or unforeseen condition that he may encounter during the procedure.

4. I consent to the administration of anesthetics to be applied by or under the direction of Dr._____ and to the use of such anesthetics and medications as he may deem advisable in my case.

5. I have been advised that the object of the operation I have requested is improvement in appearance, not perfection, that there is the possibility that imperfections might ensue, and that the results might not live up to my expectations or the goals that have

continued

been established. In this connection, I know that the practice of medicine and surgery is not an exact science and that, therefore, reputable physicians cannot guarantee results. I acknowledge that no guarantee or assurance has been made by anyone regarding the operation which I have herein requested and authorized.

6. I have been advised that part of this surgery is—may be—performed through external incisions in the skin which will leave permanent scars whose extent and location have been described to me. I have been advised that scars take one year to mature, the changes that normally occur in their appearance having been described to me.

7. I hereby give permission to Dr._____ or any assistants he may designate to take photographs for diagnostic purposes and to enhance the medical record; I agree that these photographs will remain his property. I further authorize him to use such photographs for teaching purposes or to illustrate scientific papers, books, or lectures if, in his judgment, medical research, education, or science will benefit by their use. It is specifically understood that in any such publication or use, I shall not be identified by name.

8. I understand that if Dr._____ judges at any time that my surgery should be postponed or cancelled for any reasons he may do so.

9. I hereby state that the information furnished Dr._____ during my diagnostic evaluation is correct.

10. I agree to follow the instructions given to me by Dr._____ to the best of my ability before, during, and after the above named surgical procedure.

SIGNED:_____

(patient or person authorized to give consent for the patient)

WITNESSED:_____

(not a family member)

III

Facts and Myths about Facial Plastic Surgery

8

Facelift Surgery

NONE OF US CAN ESCAPE the inexorable ticking of the biological clock. As we age, gravity, the elements, and nature all conspire against us to work unattractive changes in our skin and musculature.

While men traditionally have accepted these changes as inevitable, women have not been so willing to compromise. For centuries they have looked to magic cures and creams in vain, hoping to hold Mother Nature at bay. More recently, first for the wealthy and then for the less well-to-do who consider it a personal investment—not a luxury—women and men have turned to the facial plastic surgeon for a safe, more effective remedy: the facelift. Facelifts are the most common facial plastic surgery procedure for reducing the signs of aging, and often are performed in conjunction with other procedures such as the chemical peel, eyelid surgery, and the eyebrow lift.

One such person is Maye Keao of Mobile, Ala. "I knew I would look better, but I didn't know it would be this much better," Maye explains with a note of exaltation in her voice. "I was well prepared for the surgery by my surgeon, so I knew about all the possible problems. But I wasn't prepared for how great I would look."

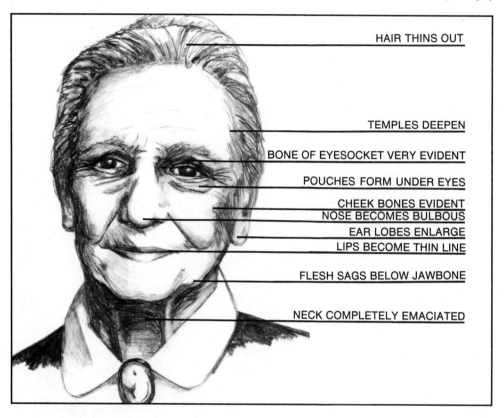

HAIR THINS OUT

TEMPLES DEEPEN

BONE OF EYESOCKET VERY EVIDENT

POUCHES FORM UNDER EYES

CHEEK BONES EVIDENT
NOSE BECOMES BULBOUS
EAR LOBES ENLARGE
LIPS BECOME THIN LINE

FLESH SAGS BELOW JAWBONE

NECK COMPLETELY EMACIATED

''Everybody has told me that I look 15 years younger,'' she adds. ''It's just wonderful.''

Maye is one of many men and women who have learned of the dramatic difference a facelift can make in their lives. Says a facial plastic surgeon from Birmingham, Ala., ''We're seeing a tremendous increase in the number of both men and women seeking facelifts. And today, fully 10 percent of all facelifts are performed on men, a significant increase from just 10 years ago.''

With age, the skull becomes smaller, and some of the fat pads in the face are absorbed. The skin loses much of its elasticity and begins to sag. The muscles and tissues around the eyes weaken, causing some of the fat normally located around the eyes to bulge forward. The skin itself begins to degenerate, so it looks tired and etched with wrinkles.

What does this mean to you? You might begin to think that your skin has become too large for your face. Lines become permanently etched in your forehead and at the sides of your mouth; your eyebrows sag, bags appear under your eyes and crow's feet at their corners; jowls develop along your jawline; and a double chin appears.

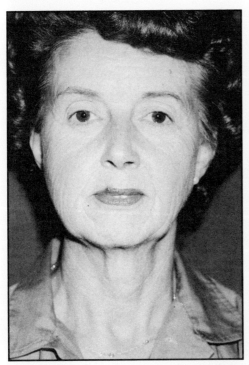 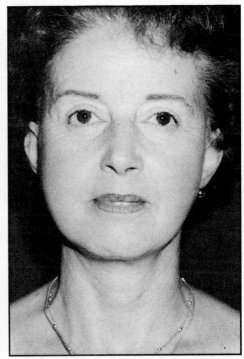

A facelift can have a dramatic effect on the signs of aging, as these before and after photos show. The smoother skin around the mouth is the result of a chemical peel, often performed in conjunction with a facelift. Eyelid surgery also was performed, but note that wrinkling still remains in the eye area. This is because a chemical peel cannot be performed at the same time as eyelid surgery.

Must all this happen to you? Probably not. "Today increasing numbers of people never want to look that bad, and they do not have to," says the surgeon from Alabama, explaining that the facelift tightens the loose skin and muscles that sag with age. ''People are having surgery performed at an earlier age than 10 or 15 years ago. In fact, many of the facelifts performed today are part of a preventive maintenance program rather than a rejuvenation effort.''

Rejuvenation or prevention: the choice is yours. If you are tired of looking in the mirror and seeing a too-old face staring back, a facelift can remove most of the sags and wrinkles and give you a face that looks five to 10 years younger. On the other hand, if you are just beginning to notice little lines and wrinkles and want to keep your youthful appearance, you may opt for a series of minor procedures to correct the signs of aging as they appear. In this way, you can remain looking younger through the years and can look forward to hearing others remark that you do not seem to grow older.

Be an Informed Patient

''It's important to know,'' says the surgeon from Alabama, ''that the word 'facelift' does not necessarily mean the same operation to every surgeon.'' Some surgeons, he explains, consider the tightening of the cheek and neck skin to be the facelift, and they may consider the forehead and the area under the chin separately. ''Patients need to be aware of this, so they can ask the right questions,'' he says.

He advises asking your surgeon exactly what the facelift includes. Will it also tighten the loose skin around the eyes, forehead, and under the chin? Does the surgery tighten muscles as well as remove loose skin? Will liposuction be used to remove fatty deposits? Will there be any extra charges for these additional procedures?

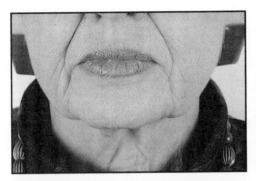
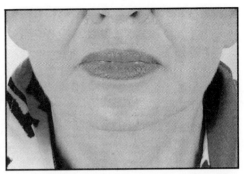

A facelift can greatly reduce jowling and reduce excess skin in the neck. The smoother skin around the mouth and the reduction of laugh lines around the mouth are a result of both the facelift and chemical peeling.

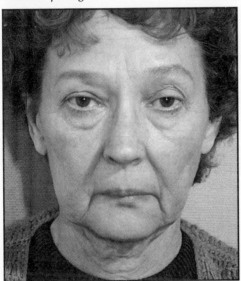
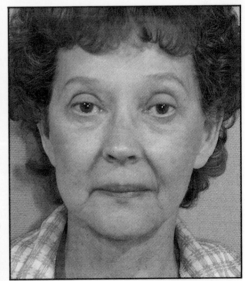

A facelift does not make the patient look younger, but rather less tired and altogether fresher.

Most people undergoing ''aging face'' surgery today choose to embark on a program of preventive maintenance before the signs of aging become too pronounced. ''The ideal time to have a first facelift,'' says an AAFPRS member, ''is before the condition gets so severe that, when surgery is performed, your friends notice a drastic change.'' But there is

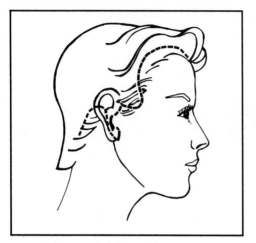

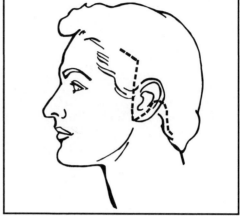

The broken lines indicate the usual location of incisions for a facelift on a woman. They are designed to be camouflaged by the hair and the natural creases around the ear.

The incisions for a facelift on a man are dictated by the pattern of beard growth and differ slightly from those made on women.

no magic age for having a facelift—only you and your surgeon can decide when it is right for you.

Part of the good news about facelifts is that the techniques are getting better year by year. ''Facial plastic surgeons are always looking for ways to improve their techniques so that the results can be more predictable and more long lasting,'' asserts that surgeon.

Facelift surgery has changed dramatically in recent years, he points out. ''Where we used to be limited to tightening the skin and removing overlapping portions, we now have methods for supporting and tightening the underlying muscles and contouring fat pads with liposuction [see chapter 17] before tightening the skin and removing the excess,'' he explains. The result? Your facelift will look better and last longer. Because of new techniques, facial plastic surgeons today can customize the facelift operation to the patient's specific needs.

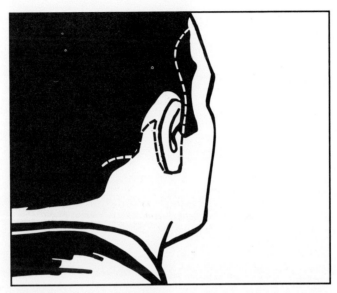

Behind the ear, the incisions on both men and women are similar. They usually are camouflaged by the natural creases in the hair.

How the Facelift Is Done

To perform a facelift, the surgeon lifts and repositions the sagging skin and underlying muscles of the face and removes some of the excess skin and fat. The incision usually begins in the temple hair above and in front of the ear, extends down in front of the ear, around the ear lobe, up behind the ear, and then backward into the hair of the scalp. For men, the incision line is altered somewhat to allow for beard growth. The skin is lifted out into the forehead, temples, cheeks, and neck; the underlying muscle and connective tissues are repositioned; and the overlapping skin is removed. Excess fat, if any, may be removed as well, and occasionally it may be necessary to make a small incision under the chin to help with the correction. Then the incisions are closed with sutures or small metal clips, which allow the surgeon to do the operation without having to shave the hair.

Misconceptions About Facelifts

I have heard that once I have a facelift, I will need to keep getting them or I'll look worse than I would have looked if I had never had the surgery in the first place. Is this true?

No. Many people have heard this myth, but it is just not true. The excessive skin that is removed in the facelift procedure never returns, although, of course, the remaining skin continues to age normally. So if a facelift makes you look 10 years younger, you will always look 10 years younger than you otherwise would have. It is true that a "tuck-up" (mini-lift), performed several years after the original facelift, can help maintain your youthful appearance by eliminating the new sagging that occurs after the facelift.

Will a facelift correct laugh and frown lines?

If these lines are visible when your face is at rest, a facelift may improve them, but chemical peeling may be necessary to achieve the best possible results. Lines that appear only during smiling and frowning are not true wrinkles and will not be affected by surgery.

Will a facelift make my skin look stretched?

The unnatural stretched or "windblown" look sometimes seen in years past after a facelift resulted from the surgeon stretching the skin too tightly and pulling it in an unnatural direction. Skillful surgeons today are able to avoid this "operated" look. Be sure to discuss your concerns with your surgeon.

Should I lose weight before surgery?

That depends. If you are committed to losing more than 20 pounds, dramatic changes in your face and body may occur with the weight loss, and you would be wise to diet sensibly first and postpone surgery until you are near your goal weight. If you plan to lose only five to 10 pounds, the changes would not be significant enough to delay surgery. Remember that crash diets tend to deplete your body of essential nutrients needed for proper healing, so you should not go on a crash diet before surgery.

When will I be presentable?

Most patients resume their preoperative routine within two weeks. Temporary swelling, discomfort, and discoloration are inevitable after a facelift, but most people find these a small price to pay for the physical and psychological improvement they experience. Cosmetics and hairstyling techniques can camouflage most of the scars and bruises as they heal.

The procedure usually takes between two and three hours. It may be performed in a hospital, an ambulatory surgical care center, or an office surgery facility. When surgery is completed, a bulky turbanlike dressing is applied, and you will be taken to a recovery area for observation.

Though facelifts can be performed safely on an outpatient basis, your surgeon may recommend a short hospital stay. If you go home shortly after your facelift, you will want to arrange to have someone available to care for you for a day or so following surgery.

The surgery itself is relatively painless. It may be done under "twilight" anesthesia, in which mild sedatives are given orally and intravenously and combined with local anesthesia, inducing "twilight sleep." Alternately, you may receive preoperative medications to relieve tension and local anesthetics to numb your face during surgery. General anesthesia may be administered if you prefer. Thoroughly discuss your questions and concerns about anesthesia with your physician in advance.

Just a Facelift?

Most people who need a facelift should consider having something done to their upper or lower eyelids, according to a facial plastic surgeon from Birmingham, Ala., who says that 90 percent of his facelift patients benefit from eyelid surgery as well.

The eyelids can be done at the same time as the facelift without increasing discomfort or recovery time (see chapter 11). On the other hand, it also is possible to have surgery done in stages, if you prefer, for economic reasons.

If your skin is very wrinkled, chemical peeling may be necessary to refine the results of your facelift. It is common for patients over the age of 50 to need chemical peeling along with their facelift (see chapter 16). Localized areas (lips, eyelids, etc.) are sometimes peeled at the same time as the facelift; but if it is necessary to peel areas that are being operated on, you must wait three months to give your facelift a chance to heal. "Peeling," says the surgeon, "is often the icing on the cake."

What About Scars?

Despite the long incision, scars resulting from facelift surgery usually are not noticeable once they have matured. Since the incision is made in hair-bearing areas and in the natural creases around and behind the ear, the scar can easily be camouflaged with hair and by the natural creases and folds around the ears.

Most surgeons do not shave any of your hair to perform the facelift. Stitches or clips are removed after one week, and much of the swelling and discoloration that follows surgery will subside within two weeks. It will take six to eight weeks for most of the swelling to disappear and for your face to reach a natural contour, but with appropriate covering cosmetics and hairstyling, you should be able to go out and follow your normal routine after about two weeks.

Your incision scars will appear quite pink after the stitches have been removed, but they can be covered with makeup, if necessary, as soon as they have closed completely and healed over. With time, the scars will whiten and become softer. The speed of healing varies, but it usually takes about a year for the scars to mature fully.

It is not uncommon to feel depressed in the weeks after surgery. ''I looked awful,'' concedes Maye Keao. ''It was amazing. The discoloration would change from hour to hour. I would look in the mirror and see my bruises move to other parts of my face, now on the left side, a couple of hours later somewhere else. There were moments when I wasn't quite sure I had made the right decision. Like when I turned that horrible chartreuse color, and I looked at myself and said 'What have I done?' But when they removed the bandage from my chin, it was great. I looked so much better, just years younger.''

A Positive Experience

"I was apprehensive before I went in, but the moment I got there all my nervousness left me," says Maye Keao four months after she had a facelift, chin implant, and chemical peel of the upper lip.

Maye remembers wanting to sleep a lot during the first two weeks after surgery. Having traveled to another city to have the surgery, she stayed for a week in an apartment provided by her surgeon. "It was like a vacation," she recalls. "My husband stayed the first couple of days, and the doctor provided a 'sitter' who stayed with me the first night and put ice bags on my face all night long." During the day, Maye took care of her incisions, fixed her own meals, and chatted with other women recovering from similar surgery.

"They wanted us to get up and be as active as possible, so the doctor provided us with a microwave and a variety of instant and easy to swallow foods," she says. "Caring for the incision involved most of my day, because the anesthesia made us clumsy and slow. My hair looked horrible. I looked horrible. But we followed the doctor's instructions carefully, putting peroxide or witch hazel on the incision and Crisco on the chemically peeled areas several times a day."

Maye and her fellow patients went to dinner at a nearby restaurant with their husbands one night. "We looked like battered wives," she laughs. Maye started going out regularly three weeks after the surgery. "Everywhere I went, people paid me compliments. Before my facelift, no one had ever told me I was pretty. Now I hear all the time how pretty I am! I love it. It took me a while to get used to all this admiration—but it was an adjustment I didn't mind making. Now I carry my 'before' picture with me, and I show it to everyone. People can't believe it.

"Everything about this was a positive experience for me."

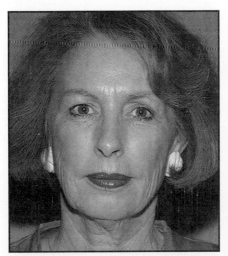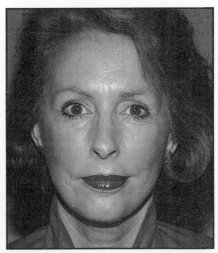

Maye Keao before and after surgery (front view)

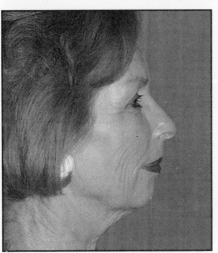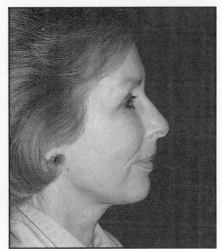

Maye Keao before and after surgery (side view)

A Personal Story

(Peter Feibleman had facelift surgery performed by a facial plastic surgeon in Beverly Hills, Calif. A professional writer, Feibleman gives this account of his procedure.)

I decided in the fall of 1987 to have surgery and made an appointment with a facial plastic surgeon. The morning of the procedure I was mildly anxious, and I asked to speak to the anesthesiologist. I was a little apprehensive since I had a history of trouble with anesthesia. I asked to be put under as completely as possible. My surgeon came in at the last moment and spoke with me, so my final memories presurgery are without anxiety of any kind.

I have no memory of the procedure itself. My first awareness was of being bandaged, and my surgeon's voice telling me it was over and everything was all right. I walked out of the operating room elated and groggy, feeling good about the whole thing.

The first night I had some mild discomfort because the bandages had been put on tight, but the nurse assured me that this was necessary and the second night would be better. She was right. The next morning the first bandages were removed and another set applied more loosely. There was no further discomfort after that.

There was no discomfort whatsoever related to the surgery, even before the first set of bandages was removed, and there was much less bruising than I had anticipated. I had spent some time at a health spa immediately preceding the surgery in order to lose weight and get in top physical shape. Partly because of that, the recovery period was shorter than I had imagined.

Within five days all bruising was gone. The swelling around my eyes lasted longer, although no one except me seemed aware of it. A week after surgery I had lunch with a friend at the hotel where I was staying, and I wore dark glasses. A week later, the glasses were no longer necessary.

In the weeks after surgery, I noticed that the swelling was up some mornings and down on others. It seemed to increase the day after I would have an alcoholic drink, so I gave up alcohol for the duration—no real hardship in my case.

It is now eight weeks since the surgery, and all residual swelling has virtually disappeared, although my surgeon told me to wait three months before expecting to see the final results.

In retrospect it seems important to have established a relationship of trust with the surgeon, to feel safe in terms of his knowledge, expertise, and taste. For a patient like me, soothing words and euphemistic talk have a reverse effect; I happen to prefer bluntness, simplicity of speech, and the truth laid out as clearly as possible.

I've seen a great many friends in the last few weeks, all of whom have told me that I look better than I have in years. No one, so far, has guessed that I had surgery, although I am not shy about letting people know. It seems to me a fine thing to have done, and the secrecy surrounding it seems foolish. I look better and therefore I feel better about myself, and so I function better in my daily life.

9

Plastic Surgery of the Nose

IF YOU HAVE EVER DESPAIRED about the size or shape of your nose, you are not alone.

"Your nose is like a signpost for everyone to see, since it is the most prominent feature on your face," points out a facial plastic surgeon who specializes in plastic surgery of the nose. "If it is out of proportion with your other features, you may feel as if it dominates your face."

"I had a terrible nose," says Mary S. "I was an athletic child, but clumsy. I had broken my nose about four times, and it just didn't suit my face."

If your nose, like Mary's, makes you unhappy because it does not do justice to your face, you do not have to live with it. Each year thousands of Americans—men and women alike—opt for nasal surgery, or rhinoplasty, as it is known in the medical profession.

Many things may be wrong with the nose you were born with. Does it have a hump on top? Has it been broken? Does it project outward too far? Is it crooked or too long, too wide, or too big for your face? Does the

A Nose Is Just a Nose

Diane S., a recent divorcée, went to a facial plastic surgeon hoping that a new nose would improve her chances of finding a replacement husband. "My wealthy parents are on my back and want me to remarry," she said.

After that declaration, the surgeon told the young woman she was expecting far too much from a rhinoplasty. "Are you happy with yourself?" he asked her. "Well, no," she replied tentatively. "I wish I could stand up to my parents."

"Perhaps you should sign up for an assertiveness course at the YWCA," the surgeon wisely suggested. "I can give you a new exterior, but the interior is your responsibility."

Diane was intelligent enough not to be offended; she knew she had a problem coping with her parents' overprotective demands. She left the surgeon's office disappointed but was back a year later to have the bridge of her nose narrowed so it would be more photogenic. It seems she did indeed take the assertiveness course—as well as one in photography—and thereby met an instructor who suggested she try modeling. She was able to secure a job as a magazine model, which boosted her self-esteem and made her parents happy as well.

Diane now wanted nasal surgery for a specific reason, and the surgeon was happy to oblige. She ended up with a finely sculpted nose that was very photogenic. Although she was very pretty to begin with, she emerged a beauty both inside and out.

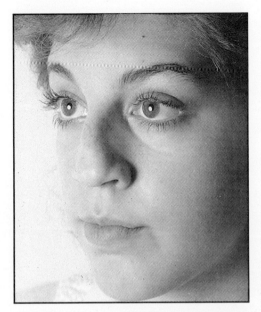 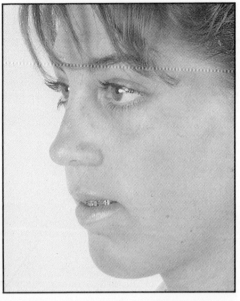

An accident when she was young caused this young woman's nose to grow crooked and deformed. Nasal surgery elevated and narrowed her tip, straightened the bridge of her nose, and made the tip of her nose come farther away from her face. The slightly different angle for three-quarter view pre- and post-operative photos was deliberately selected for this set of pictures so that the deformity and its correction would most clearly show.

tip of your nose appear big and bulbous? Or does it point downward like a hawk's bill? Whatever the problem, rhinoplasty performed by a skillful facial plastic surgeon may help to refine your nose and bring it in line with your other facial features.

If your problem goes beyond appearance—if obstructions in your nose cause difficult breathing, chronic sinus problems, or recurring headaches, you may be a candidate for septorhinoplasty, a procedure that removes internal obstructions and improves the appearance of the nose.

Perhaps your need for a new nose is more psychological. One facial plastic surgeon recalls a spry old lady in her mid-70s who came to his office to ask for a new nose. He wondered why she wanted an operation after all the years she had lived with her old nose. "Maybe you don't remember," she told the surgeon, "but some years ago you did my

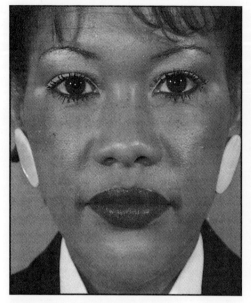 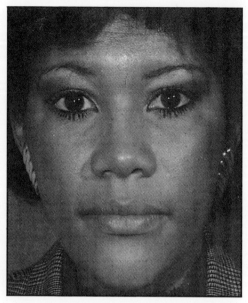

Even when there is a minor change in the nose, it makes a greatly improved and more defined facial appearance.

sister's nose. Well, she died a few months ago, and I thought she looked so good laid out that I want to have mine done so I can look just as good as she did.'' The surgeon spent some time pointing out the rigors of having surgery at such an advanced age, but the woman was adamant; she wanted to surpass her sister in just one area.

This was sibling rivalry to an extreme, perhaps. But the lady came through the surgery with flying colors and was absolutely delighted with her new nose.

Planning the Surgery

Careful planning of the rhinoplasty procedure is essential before the first incision is made. Your facial plastic surgeon probably will take a number of photographs of your nose from various angles to help him evaluate the problem and plan the procedure.

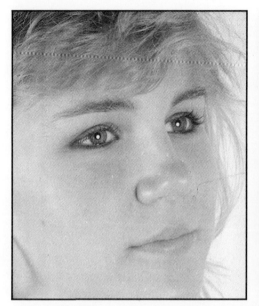 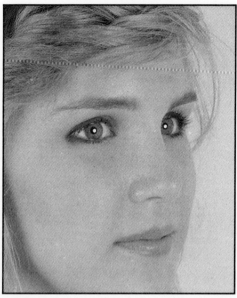

*This three-quarter profile is the best from which to see how nasal surgery can narrow a tip and,
in so doing, make the nose appear much straighter.*

"We worked on it together," says Mary S., whose nasal surgery was
a birthday gift from her husband. Her surgeon placed overlays of different noses on a photograph of her profile. Other surgeons may draw
sketches of the proposed correction or use a computer to show you what
you might look like after surgery.

"My surgery didn't give me a perfect nose," adds Mary. "My doctor explained that I didn't have a perfect face, and if I had a perfect nose
I'd look perfectly ridiculous! So he gave me a nose that was ever so slightly off center, and he left it a little bit ordinary looking. It was just perfect
for me."

The planning process will involve a thorough screening to examine
your attitudes and expectations about the surgery. You should seek
surgery because you want it, not to please others, facial plastic surgeons
advise. Surgery, they point out, can improve your profile, but it will not
change your life.

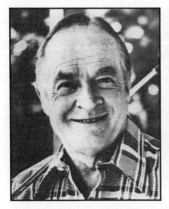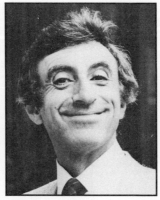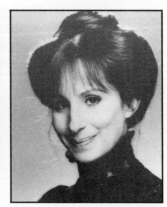

Sometimes even an imperfect nose should not be changed. Who can imagine Bob Hope, Jamie Farr, or Barbra Streisand with any noses but these? Jimmy Durante made a career based on his schnoz.

"Before I had the surgery, my nose was the first thing I noticed when I looked in the mirror," notes Mary S. "Now I never notice my nose. I think that's the real goal of facial surgery—to be able to forget your appearance. This surgery did not change my life, it just made my nose suit my face."

How Rhinoplasty Is Performed

Rhinoplasty incisions usually are hidden just inside the rim of the nostrils. To make flaring nostrils smaller, an incision may be made at the crease on the outer edge of each nostril. In more complicated cases, it may also be necessary to make a small incision between the nostrils. The cartilage and bone of the nose are reshaped through these incisions to give the nose a more pleasing appearance. The procedure takes one to two hours, depending on how much work must be done.

Rhinoplasty usually is performed under intravenous sedation with local or general anesthesia. If extensive surgery is needed, or if you are especially nervous, your surgeon may recommend general anesthesia and a short hospital stay, but rhinoplasty often is performed in an ambulatory care facility or in the surgeon's office.

Most patients report little or no pain after surgery, but postoperative discomfort can be easily controlled with mild medications. When

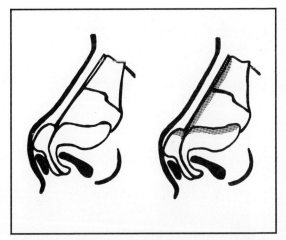

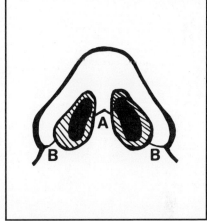

The nose is made smaller by removing excess bone and cartilage (dotted areas). The remaining structures are repositioned through a series of carefully planned internal incisions. The skin then heals to the new framework.

Incision options: **A.** The columellar incision is made in certain difficult noses. **B.** The alar incision in made when nostril width is reduced.

nasal packing is eliminated, the experience is more pleasant for the patient. A small splint usually is placed on the nose for a few days, and some kind of light internal dressing may be applied. A bulky dressing, designed to lessen swelling, may be placed on your face for a couple of hours. The internal dressing, if used, normally is removed within 24 hours, and the splint and tape after five to seven days.

Your nose probably will feel stuffy after the surgery, and you will have some swelling and discoloration. An oral decongestant may be given to ease nasal stuffiness, but you should avoid nasal sprays or drops. Swelling usually subsides quickly and continues to decrease over the next six months. Most bruising can be covered with normal makeup seven to 10 days after surgery.

"My nose looked somewhat bruised for about two or three weeks," recalls Mary. "I had yellowish bruises on my cheeks, but I went out and didn't let it bother me. I looked like someone had popped me for smarting off, but it wasn't like I had lost a three rounder!" Mary says she felt

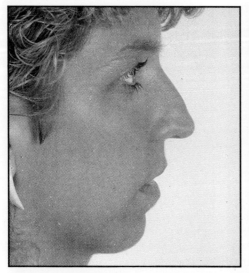 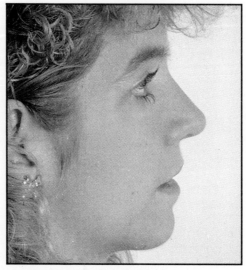

When nasal surgery is combined with a chin implant, the entire profile changes. Notice the elevation of the tip of the nose, the shortening of the nose, the straightening of the profile with increased definition of the tip, and the increased forward projection of the chin.

completely healed in three weeks, but she could not wear glasses for six weeks.

If you wear glasses, they must not put pressure on your nose during the healing process. Some patients suspend their glasses from a loop of tape to the forehead. Your surgeon may give you a special device designed to support the glasses after nasal surgery.

You may notice increased oiliness of the skin on your nose after surgery, and some patients will "break out" in whiteheads. These can be annoying but usually cause no significant problem. Thorough cleansing can help.

Occasionally, the results of the surgery may be less than satisfactory, necessitating a second procedure. A repeat operation can sometimes be more complex than the first, so it should not be taken lightly. Remember that the finished product will not be visible until months after surgery, so it is important to be patient and keep a positive attitude about your appearance.

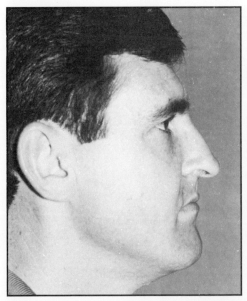 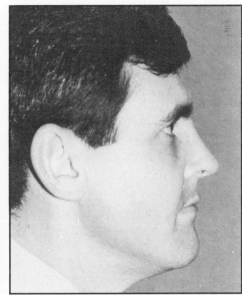

Nasal surgery is increasingly popular among men.

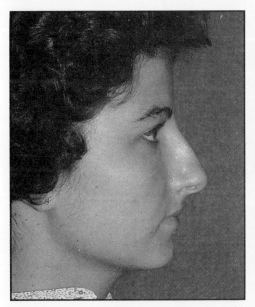 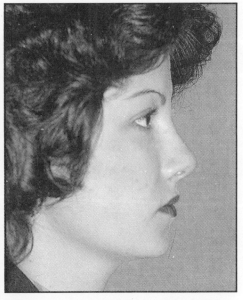

Combining nasal surgery with a direct brow lift is another possible means of improving appearance.

The cost of a rhinoplasty depends on a number of factors, including the experience and expertise of your surgeon, where you live, and the extent of your problem. Your doctor should review his fees with you well in advance.

If you need nasal surgery to correct a breathing problem, your insurance company should provide at least partial payment. You should discuss your plans with a representative of your insurance company before the surgery. Surgery that is strictly cosmetic generally is not covered by insurance.

All surgery carries some level of risk, but rhinoplasty is considered a very safe procedure. Your surgeon will thoroughly discuss risks with you before you decide on the procedure.

Nasal Surgery—What Age?

People often ask what age is best for having plastic or reconstructive surgery of the nose. Surgery may be performed on a young child with a severe breathing problem brought on by a defect of the internal structure of the nose, but additional surgery may be needed as the child matures. Explains a facial plastic surgeon from Birmingham, Ala., "There are certain limitations in performing surgery on children. It usually is not advisable to correct the problem completely before puberty."

If surgery to refine the appearance of the nose is desired, it can usually be done on girls at age 15 and on boys at age 18. There are many individual differences, however. Many surgeons advise having an initial consultation early, even if surgery is several years away, to enable the facial plastic surgeon to monitor the child's growth and development.

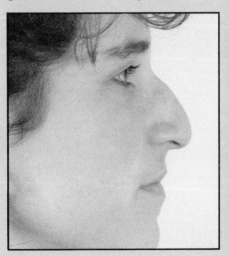 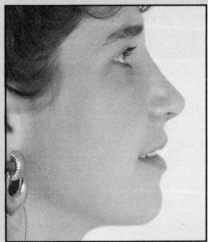

While not usually done on very young children, nose surgery is a good choice for young people in their mid-teens or older.

continued

Early correction of nasal deformities can help young people develop self-confidence and build self-esteem, but there is no upper limit to the surgery. Older patients who have been unhappy with their noses all their lives may choose surgery as long as they are in good health.

An Anniversary to Remember

Allison H. was a stylish business executive who had been happily married for 15 years. For their upcoming anniversary, her husband asked her what she would like as a gift, suggesting a cruise or a larger diamond. After giving it several days of thought, she confessed that she really wanted nasal surgery.

Her husband was not overly surprised, since he knew Allison well enough to know she had never like her flattened, scooped-up nose, but he was surprised she would pass up an exotic vacation or a precious stone for an operation. Obviously he had underestimated her desire to improve her appearance.

Allison explained to the facial plastic surgeon that she considered her nose-to-be as a present to herself, even though her husband was paying for it. As a well-paid executive, she could have paid for a rhinoplasty herself years ago, but only recently had the idea crystallized as something she really wanted.

"I was terrified that if I was put 'under,' I might not wake up," she explained. "It was not until a friend of mine had it done that I learned the anesthesia techniques of past years have been replaced with safer, outpatient methods."

Allison's facial plastic surgeon was happy to put her mind at rest about the anesthesia. He and Allison spent some time discussing how she envisioned her nose and agreed that straightening it would improve her appearance.

Her husband accompanied her on the day of the surgery and seemed more nervous than she did. She asked that the scrub nurse hold her hand during the surgery to make her feel more secure.

continued

In the recovery room, however, Allison remarked to a nurse that the "whole ordeal wasn't much of an ordeal after all."

Both Allison and her husband came to the surgeon's office for the unveiling of her new nose, and both seemed elated. Allison then turned to her husband and said she would remember this particular anniversary for the rest of her life.

10

Plastic Surgery of the Ears

ARE YOUR EARS UNEVEN, misshapen, or so large that the kindergarten crowd was wont to think up nicknames such as "elephant ears" or "Dumbo"? Physician Debbie M.'s were, and she remembers well the anguish her ears caused her.

"One thing I always hated about myself was my big ears," recalls Debbie. "I could not wear my hair behind my ears or in a ponytail, and I never wanted to go swimming because I hated to let my hair get wet. I was very self-conscious about it, especially as a teenager."

A facial plastic surgery procedure called otoplasty has made Debbie's self-consciousness a thing of the past. Today ears can be reshaped, "pinned back," and made smaller or more symmetrical—to Debbie's delight. "Now I feel a lot better about the way I look," she says. "I'm a lot more confident and I can wear my hair different ways—short, pulled back, or in a ponytail. It's really nice to have options."

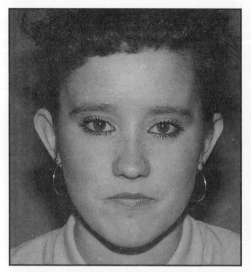 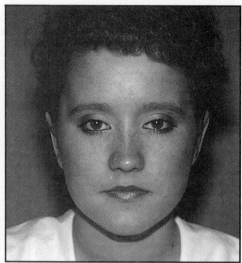

Surgery to correct protruding ears can be performed at any age, but the softer cartilage in younger patients makes it easier to mold.

Where ''Jug Ears'' Come From

Protruding ears often run in families. In some cases the development of the ears, for unknown reasons, stops short in the womb. During early prenatal (before birth) development, the ears stick straight out from the head. As the unborn baby develops, the ears usually assume a position closer to the head and develop the natural folds and convolutions of the normal ear.

If the folds do not form, the result is a cuplike ear that projects from the side of the head. Or excess cartilage may cause the ear to be too large or to sit out too far from the head.

Anyone with normally developed ears that protrude or lack symmetry may be a candidate for otoplasty, the operation that repositions or pins back protruding ears. Otoplasty also can shorten or reshape the earlobes or shorten excessively tall ears. In extreme cases—for instance, where a baby is born with no outer ear at all—advanced facial plastic surgery techniques can create a natural-looking ear.

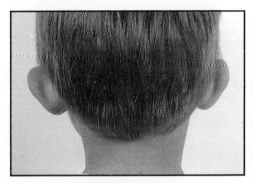 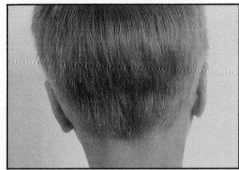

Some Big Ears Are an Asset

Not everyone with large ears will want to have them fixed—witness the success of Clark Gable. On the other hand, says an AAFPRS member who specializes in plastic surgery of the ears. ''Clark Gable's ears weren't really that bad, but they were what everyone noticed and remembered about him. He was always caricatured with tremendous, overexaggerated ears.''

People tend to be critical of unusual features, he states, and often parents may not realize how a child may feel about his or her protruding ears. Debbie M. agrees. ''My parents never suggested having it done. I wish they had gotten the surgery for me years earlier. I wanted it for years and years, ever since I was very young.'' Now a practicing physician, Debbie recommends that parents consider getting their children's protruding ears fixed early.

Otoplasty can be performed on children or adults, but the ideal time is at about 5 to 6 years of age. By this time the ear has grown to 90 percent of its adult size and is almost completely formed. Children younger than 6 generally are not aware of physical appearance, so most children of this age have not yet been subjected to the teasing and nicknames common in grade school.

Avoiding teasing is only one reason for not putting off surgery, notes one facial plastic surgeon. ''Cartilage in young children is still very soft,''

The Perfect Ear

Is there an ideal shape for ears? While ears may not be the most important beauty attribute, they definitely contribute to the overall look and balance of the face, says a facial plastic surgeon. The height of the ear should be in proportion to the rest of the face—the top of the ear at the level of the brow and the bottom of the ear in line with the base of the nose.

Ears that are out of proportion with the rest of the face can draw too much attention to themselves, marring an otherwise attractive appearance. Ears actually grow with age, becoming longer at the base.

Plastic surgery can make the earlobes smaller if they have grown unattractively long with age. On the other hand, earlobes are attracting more attention these days with our renewed interest in wearing earrings—sometimes more than one in each ear. Earlobes come in two distinct shapes: straight and attached at the side of the head, and curved and hanging. Some people don't like the shape of their earlobes, and otoplasty techniques can be used to change the shape of the earlobes.

Can the shape of the ear affect hearing? The folds and convolutions do serve to concentrate and localize sound waves, but changing the shape of the ears usually will not affect hearing. Hearing changes noticeably when a person totally loses the outer ear, but little change occurs with routine surgery to pin back or reshape the ear.

he explains. "It's good to catch the problem at that stage, before the cartilage gets too firm and cannot be molded as easily."

The operation can be done later, as Debbie will testify. But in older persons the cartilage may spring back to its former position. If this happens, a "tuck-up" procedure may need to be done later.

Some patients may have only one ear that protrudes, giving them an unbalanced look. Rarely, a patient may need surgery on only one ear, but it is usually best to operate on both sides at once to obtain the best results.

No one has ears that are exactly identical, he explains. The ears, like the rest of the face, develop separately from one another in the womb. Almost always, the right ear is a little different from the left. After successful ear surgery, the ears still may appear asymmetrical. The difference may be more evident in adults because of their stronger cartilage, but usually is not noticeable, especially if the hair is worn long. If the problem is noticeable, a second minor procedure can help.

How the Surgery is Done

Otoplasty can be performed either in a hospital or in an outpatient surgery center, depending on the age of the patient and the preference of the surgeon. Young children usually are given general anesthesia and may spend one night in the hospital. Adults may have the surgery with local anesthesia and intravenous sedation, similar to procedures done in a dentist's office.

The incision is made in back of the ear, in the crease where the ear joins the back of the head. A small amount of skin and cartilage is removed, and stitches may be placed in the cartilage to create folds that were not present before. These sutures hold the ear until the incision heals and forms scar tissue that will hold the ear in its new position.

After surgery, a soft bandage is worn for a day or two. Most people are comfortable going back to school or work within a week. Patients may be advised to wear a headband or a stocking cap for the first week after surgery, and to keep it on at night for at least two weeks.

"I had some discomfort for about a week," says Debbie, "and I found it hard to find a comfortable way to sleep, because I couldn't put pressure on my ears. The first two days were the worst, but I recovered quickly."

Few risks are involved in otoplasty. Infection may occur in some patients, but this can be prevented with antibiotics given before surgery and for several days after. Other than the slight possibility that a second "tuck-up" procedure may be needed, there are usually no complications.

The Look You Want

The goal of the otoplasty procedure is a natural looking ear, facial plastic surgeons emphasize. Done correctly, there should be no surgical or "operated on" appearance. While few functional reasons for otoplasty exist—poorly shaped ears usually hear as well as perfect ones—the surgery can provide dramatic cosmetic benefits. "My protruding ears kept me from looking the way I really wanted to look," says Debbie M. "Now, after surgery, the real me can come out."

Some people choose to have otoplasty incorporated into a facelift (see chapter 8), which also involves an incision behind the ear. Attractively positioned ears can build self-esteem and make the patient feel more confident. Debbie agrees. "I didn't tell people about my surgery right away," she says, "but lately I'm telling people. I feel great about it!"

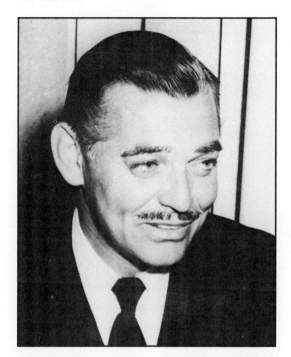

Not everyone will feel a need to have his ears adjusted, even when they're obviously large or asymmetrical. Clark Gable is a case in point.

11

Plastic Surgery of the Eyelids

THE EYES HAVE BEEN CALLED the windows of the soul. we use them to convey a wealth of emotions and to reflect our deepest feelings.

But what if your eyes project a message that is not what you feel? Are droopy, hooded upper lids telling the world that you are stern, remote, or even angry? Do puffy bags under your eyes make you look tired, dreary, or just plain old? If so, you have plenty of company.

"Eyelid surgery is the second most common procedure I do," says a facial plastic surgeon from Houston, Texas. "The skin around the eyes is one of the first things to go as we age. Many people are only in their 30s or 40s when they first notice that baggy eyes are making them look tired and older than they are."

Blepharoplasty is the medical term for the procedure that removes excess skin from the upper eyelid or protruding fatty tissue from the lower eyelid. Upper and lower lids can be treated at the same time, and the procedure also can be done in conjunction with nasal surgery (see chapter 9) or a facelift (see chapter 8).

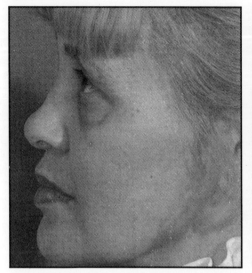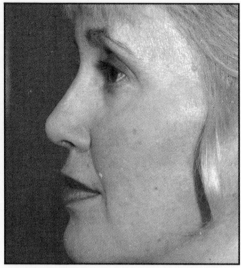

Lower eyelid surgery can be combined with nasal surgery for a more youthful appearance. In this case, the bridge of a "saddle" nose was built up with a plastic material.

For many people, according to the surgeon from Texas, blepharoplasty (also called an eyelid lift) is the first step toward rejuvenating an aging face. Long before a full facelift becomes necessary—perhaps in the 40s or 50s—an individual may wish to begin reversing the signs of aging with blepharoplasty.

"My eyelids were overhung," says Bob Damkroger of Houston, Texas, as he describes how he looked before having a blepharoplasty. "They were so overhung that it actually affected my vision. The surgery helped me to see better as well as look better."

Increasing numbers of both men and women are having blepharoplasty today. More than 100,000 people each year choose surgery to permanently eliminate excess skin and puffy bags under their eyes. "Women tend to notice the problem earlier, because they begin to have trouble applying makeup," says a facial plastic surgeon from Minnesota. "Athletes, both men and women, sometimes notice their eyelids sticking slightly when they blink while perspiring. Men typically come in when

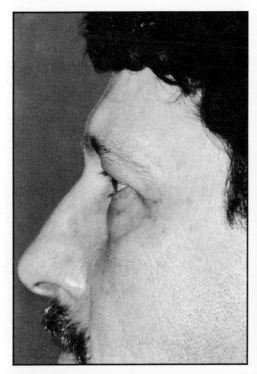 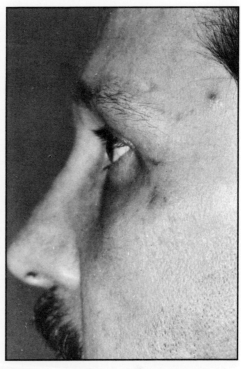

Notice how the upper lid hooding and lower lid bags were improved through facial plastic surgery.

the problem is more advanced, usually because of baggy lower lids or obstructed vision when they look up.''

Eyelid surgery, especially when combined with an eyebrow lift (see chapter 14), can dramatically open the entire upper third of the face, giving a fresher, more youthful appearance and a brighter outlook on life.

''The surgery did not change my looks,'' comments Damkroger. ''It just made me look more relaxed.''

Upper Eyelid Problems

Each time you blink—something you do billions of times over the course of your lifetime—the skin and muscles of your upper eyelids stretch a tiny bit. Elastic fibers in the skin cause them to snap back, but

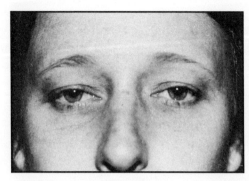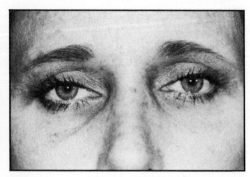

A more youthful appearance may be obtained through upper eyelid surgery, which improves the natural contours of the upper eyelid and removes excessive skin.

eventually the skin and muscles of the upper eyelids actually get longer. Excess skin may even form a hood over the eyelid.

If you have allergies or have had several pregnancies—conditions that cause the eyelids to swell—you may be more prone to developing thick, overhanging upper eyelids. If saggy eyelids run in your family, if you receive excess exposure to the sun, or if you habitually squint a lot, your upper eyelids are likely to sag as you age. This condition can occur even in relatively young people.

Excess upper eyelid skin may interfere with your vision if it overlaps too much and forms a hood over your lid, actually resting on your eyelashes. If your doctor determines that your upper lids are obstructing your vision, corrective surgery may be covered by your insurance plan.

Sagging Lower Lids

Puffy, baggy lower eyelids are a telltale sign of aging—and a distressing one because the problem is nearly impossible to hide. Furthermore, almost everyone develops some degree of bagginess under the eyes with time.

The eye is surrounded with fatty tissue encased in a membrane that tightly holds it next to the eye. This membrane weakens as it ages, and the fat begins to protrude. This stretches the skin and muscle of the lower eyelid and causes noticeable bulges.

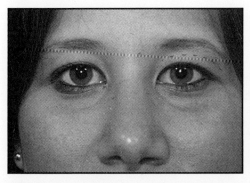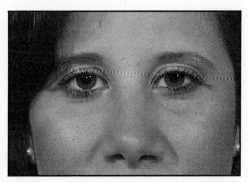

This is an example of the younger person who has a hereditary problem with droopy eyelid folds that obscure the eyelid. The condition makes application of cosmetics difficult and ineffective.

"It's not always a sign of age," adds the surgeon from Minnesota. Heredity is a big factor. Bags often occur in young people, too, and since they only get worse with age, it can be a good idea to have the problem dealt with early.

The fatty tissue around the eye can hold a considerable amount of water. When you lie down to sleep, the protruding fat absorbs extra fluid. When you awake, your eyelids may appear puffy until gravity draws the extra fluid away. The more fatty tissue you have protruding, the more your lower eyelids swell and the longer it takes to clear up. While creams and lotions may make the skin of the lower eyelids appear smoother temporarily, no cosmetic product will treat the underlying cause of puffy eyelids.

"This surgery is designed to get rid of bags," reminds the surgeon from Minnesota. "It may tighten the skin a little, but it is not intended to get rid of wrinkles." Everyone has some wrinkles under the eyes. A little looseness is needed there to smile, frown, and express other emotions. If there is excess wrinkling under the eyes, a chemical peel may be advised several weeks or months after eyelid surgery (see chapter 16).

The Mechanics of Blepharoplasty

During a blepharoplasty, excess skin in the upper lid is removed through an incision made in the natural crease above the eye. Protruding fatty tissue in the lower lid usually is removed through an incision just below the lower eyelid. The resulting scars are quite inconspicuous when healed. Women can completely camouflage any remaining marks with eye makeup. Most men find that the scars disappear into their natural ''smile'' lines.

Eyelid surgery usually is performed in an ambulatory surgical center or an office surgery facility. Local anesthesia, along with medication to help you relax, generally is used.

After surgery, the facial plastic surgeon may place small sterile strips over the incisions to help keep them closed. Your eyes may not be covered, but your surgeon may ask you to place an ointment in your eyes that will make your vision a little blurry for a day or so. The ointment helps keep the eyes from drying out. Your eyelids will be swollen, and you may be unable to close them entirely for several days after surgery, but you will be able to sleep. If you have any discomfort after surgery, it can be easily controlled with mild medications. Swelling and bruising will subside quickly if you use cold compresses and elevate your head when you lie down.

Most people are able to return to their normal routine within seven to 10 days after surgery. It may help to wear dark glasses for a few days, both to cover the swelling and to remind you not to touch your eyelids while they heal. If you wear contact lenses, you must wait two to three weeks before you can resume wearing them.

Feeling good and looking good have a lot in common. If people constantly treat you as if you are weary and tired when you feel vital and energetic, it eventually can affect the way you feel. Comments Bob Damkroger: ''I didn't expect to look 24 again because I'm almost 55. I did it because it makes me feel good.''

Permanent Lashliner

Imagine never having to apply eyeliner again. Now it is possible to have permanent eyeliner applied by a facial plastic surgeon. The procedure involves placing tiny dots of permanent pigment just below the surface of the skin at the lashline. Several different colors are available, and a skillful surgeon will apply the liner in a way that best enhances the shape of your eyes. The effect is natural looking, and the liner does not wash off.

Lashliner sometimes can be placed at the same time that a blepharoplasty is done, says a facial plastic surgeon who practices in Houston, Texas. "Permanent lashliner is not as popular as some other facial plastic surgery procedures, but it works well and is relatively safe."

Permanent lashliner actually is a type of tattooing. Other forms of tattooing used in facial plastic surgery include lip lining and lip reconstruction, which may be performed after a lip tumor is excised. Lashliner is just one of many new developments in facial plastic surgery. It is not widely used but may be indicated in limited situations.

Many women can benefit from the cosmetic convenience of permanent lashliner: women who wear bifocals or contact lenses, women with arthritis or other problems that make it difficult to apply eye makeup, women allergic to eye makeup, and women who frequently engage in active sports such as swimming or jogging, as well as working women who have little time to devote to applying makeup.

Functional reasons also exist for having the procedure. Women with scarred or altered eyelid margins and people who

continued

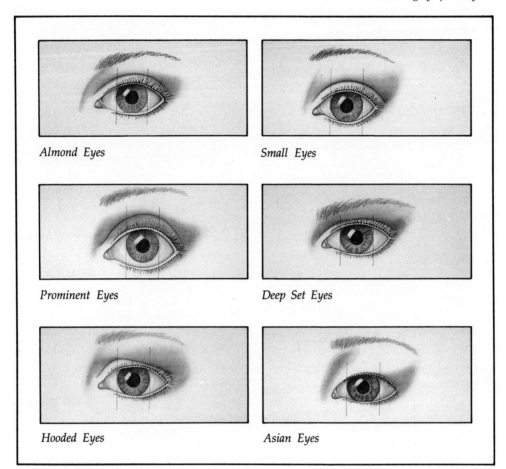

Almond Eyes

Small Eyes

Prominent Eyes

Deep Set Eyes

Hooded Eyes

Asian Eyes

have had lash loss due to trauma, lid reconstruction, or burns are good candidates. None of the therapies for lash loss work very well, and permanent lashliner can camouflage the problem. Based on the principle that light colors make things visually more prominent and dark colors make objects seem to recede, the lashliner can make prominent eyes appear smaller or close-set eyes further apart.

Corrective cosmetic consultant Susan Cristian of Sacramento, Calif., has identified six basic eye shapes and suggested placement of pigment for optimal effect as shown at left.

12

Plastic Surgery of the Chin and Jaw

WHEN GERRY RUSSO looked in the mirror each morning, the first thing he saw was his nose, which had been broken several times. He never noticed his chin because, basically, he did not have one.

Because of the multiple breaks, a deviated septum (congenital malformation of the wall between the nasal passages), and chronic sinus problems, Russo assumed his facial plastic surgery would involve only nasal surgery (see chapter 9). But his surgeon suggested a chin implant, which could be done at the same time his nose was corrected.

"He showed me what a normal face is supposed to look like," Russo recalls of his consultation with the facial plastic surgeon. "I went home and looked at anatomy books and drawings by people like Michelangelo and Leonardo da Vinci. All the men had strong, prominent chins. So I decided to go ahead and do it."

The result? "I'm so happy with the way it came out. I definitely would recommend this to anyone."

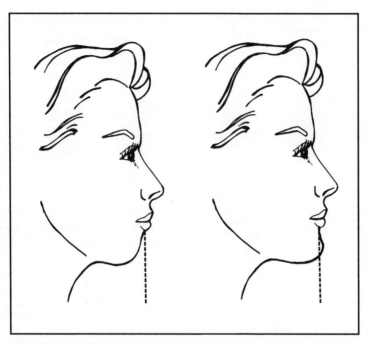

From the lower lip, a line extended straight down will fall in front of a receding chin, but cut through a protruding chin.

Russo's experience is not unusual, according to a facial plastic surgeon from Miami Beach, Fla. "Noses attract a great deal of attention," he says, "but few people go to a facial plastic surgeon because of a weak chin." Facial balance, he notes, is the key. "Your nose may seem too prominent because of its position on your face and its relationship to other facial features. A well-shaped nose can appear unattractively large on a face with a sloping forehead and a receding chin."

Does a weak chin make your other facial features seem out of balance? If so, a chin implant—or augmentation mentoplasty—may be part of the solution. Chin implants often are done along with nasal surgery (chapter 9), facelifts (chapter 8), and other facial procedures. "More than 30 percent of the people who come to me for nasal surgery also need their chins built up, and most of them do not realize that their weak chins contribute to the problem," says the surgeon from Florida.

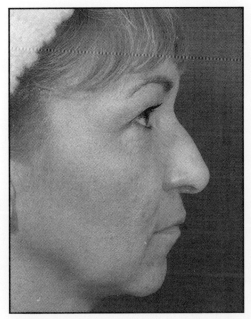 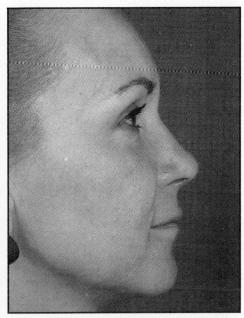

A chin implant, along with nasal and upper eyelid surgery, can make the profile more pleasing.

On the other hand, your chin may protrude excessively because of an abnormally large "chin button," or it may have become unattractively long with age. The solution? Reduction mentoplasty—a technique for removing excess bony tissue from the chin—may help you achieve a more pleasing appearance. Both procedures can yield dramatic benefits in individuals with a receding or protruding chin who have a normal jawline and dental bite.

When the problem is more severe (for example, if structural abnormalities or dental malocclusions are present), up-to-date surgical techniques (orthognathic surgery) can not only improve the function of your teeth, jaws, and other facial structures, but can do wonders for your appearance as well.

Mentoplasty: A Minor Procedure With Major Results

"It's great when a relatively minor procedure can make a truly dramatic difference in a person's appearance," says the facial plastic surgeon from Florida. "That's what makes the chin implant one of my favorite procedures. When done in conjunction with other facial plastic surgery, it only takes about 15 minutes longer. But it can make a tremendous difference in the balance of the facial features."

Chin surgery, he explains, adds little to the cost and length of the operation and does not significantly increase the risk. Many patients initially are opposed to having anything done to their chins. "In reality," says the surgeon from Florida, "though it seems like additional surgery, it enables us to do less to the nose and achieve better results. We can make the nose seem smaller relative to the other features of the face if the chin is in proper balance."

Christina Lorences, one of his patients, agrees. "I don't really have a small nose," she says, "but with the chin surgery, it balances out more. I used to be very self-conscious about my profile. I would turn away if someone was alongside me. Now my profile is great!"

To perform a chin implant, the surgeon makes a small incision either inside the mouth, between the lower lip and gum, or in the small crease under the chin. The healed scar is scarcely visible. Local anesthesia and mild intravenous sedation are most often used, although you may receive stronger anesthesia if you are having more than one procedure done at the same time.

"The surgeon creates a small pocket," explains the facial plastic surgeon from Florida, "and slips the implant into place. Then the incision is sutured, and a small dressing is placed on the chin for a few days." Implants come in several shapes and sizes, enabling the facial plastic surgeon to select one that will give a natural appearance. They are made from semisolid, spongelike, or mesh synthetic materials that closely mimics the feel of natural body tissues.

Nasal Surgery or Chin Implant?

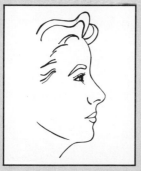 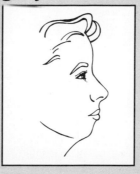 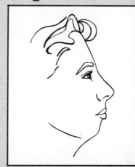

Do you really need nasal surgery? Other facial features can make your nose appear more prominent than it really is. The noses in these three profiles are identical. The face on the left, showing normal jaw structure, presents a pleasing appearance. Notice how the nose appears more prominent when the chin recedes (middle). When a long sloping forehead is combined with the weak chin (right), the nose seems to project even more.

Chin reduction surgery is performed in a similar way. The incision usually is made beneath the chin, where the scar will be hidden in a natural fold, and an instrument much like a dental drill is used to shave off a small amount of excess bony tissue. In some cases, it is necessary to make an incision inside the mouth and slide a portion of the jawbone under the roots of the teeth.

After mentoplasty, you should expect to feel a good deal of tenderness in your chin during the first few days, but any real discomfort usually is easily controlled. "I had no pain during the procedure," recalls Gerry Russo, who had both a rhinoplasty and chin augmentation. "My chin hurt worse than my nose, and I took pain medication for a day after surgery. I was a little uncomfortable, but it was not too bad, and certainly not the worst surgery I've had."

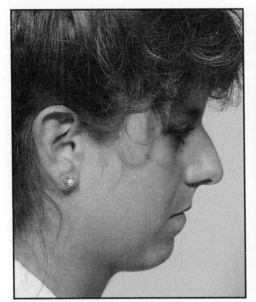 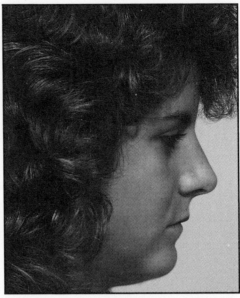

Many patients think they need only nose reduction surgery, when in fact a small chin implant can enhance surgery.

You will have to remain on a diet of liquids and soft foods for the first week to 10 days, since excess chewing may stress the area and cause the implant to shift. Your chin may look too large and feel strangely stretched for a few days after surgery, but six weeks later you will feel normal and most of the swelling will be gone. You can resume most normal activities a week to 10 days after surgery, but you should wait a bit longer before engaging in strenuous athletics or contact sports.

You may find it difficult at first to get used to your new chin. ''I doubted my chin implant for a time,'' says Christina Lorences wryly. ''It made my mouth look funny, and people would ask what was wrong with my mouth. But my doctor encouraged me to bear with it. Sure enough, as the swelling went down my face looked better.

''People now say I look great,'' she adds. ''Most people never guess what's different about me unless I tell them. I feel really good about this. I'm glad I did it.''

Who Needs Orthognathic Treatment?

If you have a handicapping malocclusion, where the teeth are so poorly aligned that their function is compromised or the teeth, jaws, or facial joints are in danger of degeneration, you may be a candidate for orthognathic treatment. Some examples:

- *Excessive overbite* (upper teeth that project too far forward), perhaps accompanied by a tendency to show too much of the upper gums even while the mouth is at rest.
- *Difficulty keeping the lips together*, which may cause mouth breathing and lead to periodontal disease.
- *Underbite*, or a lower jaw that projects forward with lower teeth in front of upper teeth.
- *An extremely underdeveloped lower jaw*, leading to an extremely receding chin and badly aligned teeth.
- *TMJ syndrome*, or pain resulting from misalignment of the joint immediately in front of the ears.
- *Bruxism* (the tendency to clench and grind the teeth while asleep), when caused by poor relationship of the jaws and teeth, which can lead to severe damage if untreated.

"I like the way it brings out the features of my face," comments Gerry Russo. "Having the surgery has really boosted my self-confidence. It is definitely worth the little bit of discomfort I experienced."

Repairing Structural Abnormalities

What if your problem is not your chin, but a jawbone that is either too long or underdeveloped? Or perhaps your teeth have never fit together properly. Structural problems of the jaws, teeth, and face can

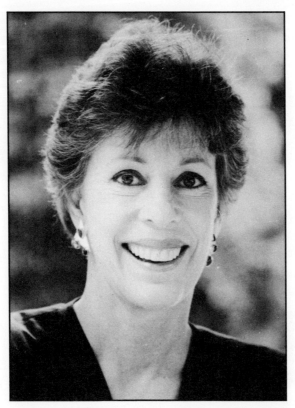

Entertainer Carol Burnett had her lower jaw and teeth brought forward through orthodontics and orthognathic surgery.

cause problems with appearance and interfere with the functions of facial structures—chewing, swallowing, smelling, seeing, and speaking.

The techniques for correcting such problems are called orthognathic surgery. The treatment requires close cooperation between the patient's dentist, orthodontist, and surgeon. Orthodontic treatment (braces) often is needed both before and after surgery.

The process begins with diagnosis of facial and skeletal abnormalities and formulation of a treatment plan. This requires a physical exam, dental models, x-rays, and prediction tracings. Then orthodontic treatment

Is Chin Surgery for You?

"I often see patients who have had a rhinoplasty [nose surgery] but who still feel that something is missing," says a facial plastic surgeon from Miami Beach, Fla. A chin implant may provide that missing something. Here is an easy way to tell if you might benefit from surgery to build up or reduce your chin.

Look at your profile in a mirror, or examine it in a photograph. Imagine a line that drops straight down from your lower lip. The tip of your chin should just touch this line. If your chin slopes back from the line, augmentation mentoplasty can improve your appearance and may even be required if you are having nasal surgery. If your chin extends beyond the line, you might benefit from chin reduction surgery.

Your surgeon will examine a number of factors, including your overall size, the size and position of your nose, how far your nose protrudes relative to the rest of your face, the alignment of your jaws, and the position of your teeth. He is the best person to advise you whether your chin is fine or you are a candidate for simple augmentation or reduction mentoplasty or whether you need more extensive surgery.

is begun to align the teeth in the jaws to accommodate the new jawbone positions provided by the surgery. This preparatory phase may take anywhere from six months to one-and-a-half years.

The surgery itself is best performed after the adolescent growth spurt when the facial skeleton is approaching its adult size. Orthodontic treatment usually is started before this time. It may take from one to two years to complete the entire process.

Most incisions in orthognathic surgery are made within the mouth, so there are usually no perceptible scars. The upper or lower jaw or both are freed from their attachments and repositioned. Then the jaw is secured in its proper position with wires, plates, or screws, and the incisions are closed with resorbable (dissolving) stitches.

The surgery usually takes place in the hospital under general anesthesia and requires a two- or three-day stay. Swelling and bruising should be expected after surgery and may take a month or more to subside completely, but most patients are presentable about a week after surgery and can resume daily activities. A liquid diet is necessary at first, though most patients can begin chewing about two weeks after surgery. Healing usually takes place rapidly.

The cost of orthognathic surgery varies depending on the extent of the work required. The surgeon's fee can range from $1,000 to $4,000 if the surgery is limited to one jaw, and twice that if both jaws are involved. There may also be fees for the services of an anesthesiologist and for the use of the hospital facility. Insurance may cover some of these costs, particularly if the surgery is intended to correct a functional problem.

13

Plastic Surgery of the Cheeks

AS WE HAVE SEEN, that elusive concept of ideal beauty is based on a harmony of facial contours. One of the chief elements of that facial harmony is the presentation and positioning of the cheekbones.

Every aspiring fashion model—and millions of women who simply wish they looked like one—understands the importance of cheekbones, especially those that are sufficiently prominent. One facial plastic surgeon simply puts it this way: "Everyone looks better with cheekbones."

Most women agree. Great cheekbones make Linda Evans and Brooke Shields look the way they do, and makeup cannot always provide what nature has omitted. Certainly not every woman should have surgery just to add cheekbone definition to her face. But if undeveloped cheekbones give your face a flat contour, you may benefit from a procedure called malar augmentation or, more simply, cheek implants.

"I always felt I had a really narrow face, and my facial features did not stand out," comments Terri Hoffman of Miami, Fla. "That's why I wanted cheek surgery—to add some definition to my face."

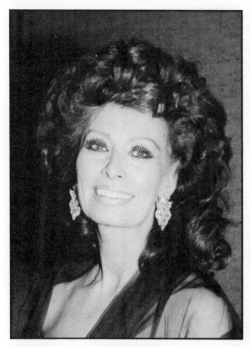 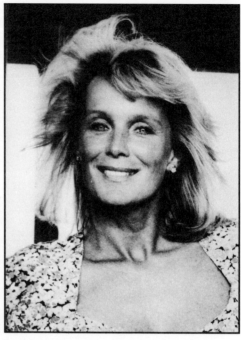

Sophia Loren (left) and Linda Evans have cheekbones that are the envy of many women.

Malar augmentation also can give the face a more youthful appearance and can improve facial harmony by deemphasizing a prominent nose or projecting chin. That is why cheek implants frequently are performed along with other facial plastic surgery procedures as part of a coordinated program of corrective surgery.

"The malar augmentation procedure—if the patient is appropriately selected and the procedure correctly applied with an appropriate implant—can be very rewarding to the patient," notes a facial plastic surgeon from Santa Rosa, Calif.

More than Skin Deep

Not everyone is a candidate for malar augmentation. Among the problems is the positioning of the implant. Much advance consideration must accompany the insertion of the implant so that the resulting cheek

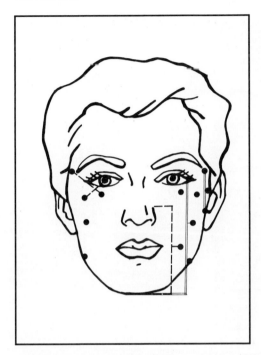

Facial plastic surgeons evaluate the relationship among the six points shown above when determining whether a patient might benefit from cheek implants and, if so, where to place the implant.

contour enhances the face and doesn't simply add an unpleasing lump. Before deciding on surgery, your surgeon will analyze your face, take a number of photographs from different angles, and thoroughly explore your motivation for having the surgery and your expectations about the results.

According to the surgeon from California, it is important to understand that even among those people with pleasing cheekbones, there is a great difference in the structure of the malar mound—the term he uses to describe the contour of the lateral face and the midface. Because of these differences, not everyone is a candidate for this kind of surgery.

A long-distance runner, for example, who basically has no subcutaneous (under the skin) fat, would be a terrible candidate for malar augmentation ''because what you are going to do is convert a flat face to a face with a small lump on it,'' the facial plastic surgeon from California says. ''Many things go into the malar mound in addition to just the bone and the soft tissue,'' he continues. ''You have to understand the

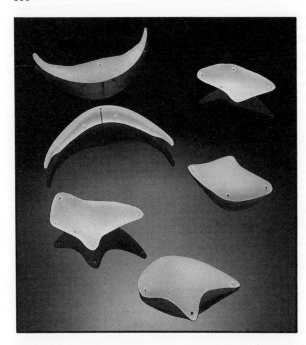

Cheek and chin implants (see chapter 12) come in a variety of sizes and shapes.

contour points. You have to understand where you want the malar eminence—the most prominent segment of the implant. A lump on the face is not necessarily attractive.''

This particular facial plastic surgeon uses a computer to analyze the face according to a set of reference points he uses to define the malar mound. Some surgeons actually draw lines on the face to determine the proper placement of the implant.

Kinds of Implants

The implant itself is made of medical grade plastic, usually of approximately triangular shape. A number of different types of implants are available; different surgeons have different preferences.

The surgeon from Santa Rosa, Calif., for example, uses a composite implant with a serrated backing that contours to the bone much like the backing of a rubber bath mat. The segment of the implant that runs along the front of the cheek is difficult for patients to feel and find.

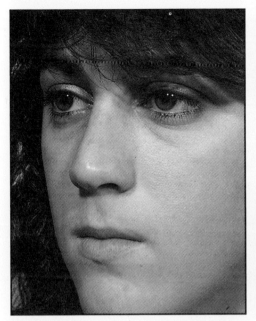 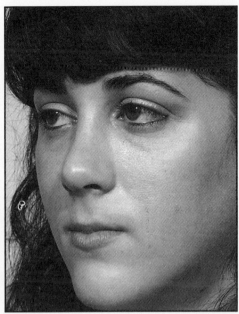

"I wanted cheek surgery to add some definition to my face," says Terri Hoffman.

Surgical Placement

The incision used for placing the implant may be made either inside the mouth or just below the lower eyelids. Most surgeons favor the internal approach, which seems to present the fewest problems for patients. The incision is made between the upper gums and the cheek, the soft cheek tissue is elevated, and a pocket is created over the cheekbone. The implant is slid through the incision and held with sutures, which are removed after six days.

The external approach uses an incision identical to that used for a lower eyelid tuck. In fact, the surgery may be done at the same time as eyelid surgery (see chapter 11). If this approach is used, the scar eventually fades to a scarcely visible line beneath the lower lashes.

Local anesthetics with mild intravenous sedation usually are preferred for cheek implants. The surgery generally is performed in the surgeon's office or in an outpatient surgery center. After surgery, you will be transferred to a recovery area to rest and recover from the sedation before being taken home.

Your face will be somewhat swollen for about two weeks after surgery, and it may be difficult to chew. You may experience some tightness or numbness around your cheeks that will feel strange while shaving or kissing. Your surgeon may suggest not brushing the teeth closest to the incision for several days, although you can use a mild mouthwash. There usually is not much discoloration after a cheek implant, and you should be able to eat ordinary food afterward without any problems.

"I was really swollen in the beginning," Terri Hoffman says. "After about six to nine months, I could really see a difference. Everything is fine now. I like the way my face looks now, much better than before. It has made me feel better about myself."

Few complications are associated with cheek implants. Of course, all surgery contains some element of risk. Your surgeon will thoroughly discuss all the risks with you well in advance of the surgery.

Is it worth it? Says Hoffman, "I like it. I don't have any regrets about having it done. I was kind of nervous at first because I didn't know what to expect, but I am glad I decided to do this."

The difference in her appearance, though subtle, is important, Hoffman explains. "People who see me do not know that I have had it done, but I feel more confident. I don't feel bad about myself anymore. I no longer feel ugly."

14

Plastic Surgery of the Forehead and Eyebrows

ALL SKIN LOSES elasticity as it ages. Add to this the effects of gravity, and what you may get is a wrinkled forehead and heavy eyebrows that push down against your upper eyelids, making your eyes look small and tired. If you also have excess skin on your upper eyelids, the combination can have a dramatic effect on your appearance—and your feelings.

"My eyebrows were starting to droop, and my eyes looked as if they were getting smaller," says Barbara Tracey when asked what prompted her to consult a facial plastic surgeon. "I seemed to look tired all the time."

"I first noticed that I had trouble putting on eye shadow, and my eyeliner kept getting on the upper part of my eyelids," she continues. This is one of the first noticeable signs of aging in women, according to

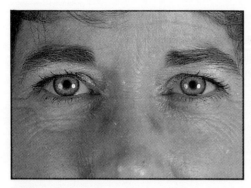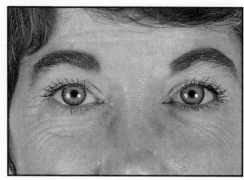

Barbara Tracy before and after eyebrow lift surgery.

a facial plastic surgeon from Omaha, Neb. Others do not realize the problem until they find themselves looking through their eyelashes.

Consider the Forehead Lift

If your problem is droopy or heavy eyebrows, a permanently furrowed brow, or a tense, angry look that does not go away, a forehead lift may be able to help.

During this procedure, an incision is made across the top of the head in the hairline. The forehead and brows are lifted and redraped upward, and the resulting excess skin is removed. The scar is hidden in the hairline.

A forehead lift not only raises your eyebrows, but also eases deep furrows between your eyes and the long horizontal lines across the forehead. It also can diminish excess smile lines at the outer corners of your eyes.

Direct—or Midforehead—Eyebrow Lift

Men are even more likely than women to have eyebrows that droop with time, but the forehead lift is not always advisable because of the difficulty in hiding the scar on a man whose hairline may later recede. For men, the recommended treatment for sagging eyebrows is the eyebrow lift.

Why Wait?

Droopy eyebrows are a common symptom of aging but can occur in younger people as well. Overhanging eyebrows and deeply furrowed forehead skin are sometimes the result of heredity.

"Even younger people can benefit from a forehead or eyebrow lift if they naturally have low eyebrows," says a facial plastic surgeon from Nebraska. "If the eyebrows are droopy to begin with, they will only get worse as a person ages."

Eyebrow surgery generally is performed on people in their 40s and 50s, when the signs of aging are just beginning to show. But you need not wait until the problem is well developed. If your eyes seem hooded by heavy, overhanging brows; or if the face you present to the world looks stern, tired, angry, or sad—no matter what your age—you may find the benefits of surgery are a fair trade for the cost and risks.

"I wanted to have it done early, so I could have years to enjoy the results," says Barbara Tracey. "Why wait until I really look old?"

During an eyebrow lift, the incision is made above the eyebrows, often in a natural forehead wrinkle, and a wedge-shaped section of excess skin is removed from above the drooping eyebrows. The underlying muscles may be supported by permanent sutures.

Sometimes the incision may be placed directly across the forehead. This procedure is called a midforehead lift. It is most often recommended for men, who have an abundance of natural forehead wrinkles that hide the scar.

Women, too, can have a direct eyebrow lift. The scar is a narrow line just above the eyebrow hairs, easily camouflaged with makeup. "I have

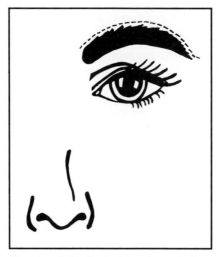

*Here is where the incision is made for a
direct brow lift.*

a rather high hairline, so my doctor recommended a direct eyebrow lift,"
Barbara Tracey explains. "The scar is not really noticeable, and I don't
do anything special to hide it." A direct eyebrow lift also may be appropriate for a woman if her eyebrows are asymmetrical and only one
needs to be raised, or if the eyebrows are very droopy and need to be
raised quite a distance.

Little Discomfort Noted

Eyebrow lifting can be performed painlessly and comfortably under
local anesthesia with "twilight sleep" sedation, and usually no
hospitalization is required; the procedure most often is performed in an
office surgery facility or ambulatory surgical center.

Little discomfort is associated with eyebrow lifting. Routine swelling and bruising subside in a week to 10 days and can be hidden with
makeup as soon as your incisions heal. You can return to work as soon
as you feel up to it, usually within one to two weeks, although you should
avoid strenuous physical activities for at least three weeks.

If you have severe drooping of the eyelids caused by sagging eyebrows and excess upper eyelid skin, your peripheral vision may be impaired. If this is the case, the procedure has a functional basis and may be covered by your insurance. Your doctor may have you see an ophthalmologist or optometrist for a visual field examination to test your peripheral vision. The results of that examination and photographs of your eyes are then sent to your insurance company to determine whether coverage is appropriate.

Other Procedures

Eyebrow or forehead surgery may be done alone if droopy eyebrows or a furrowed forehead is your only problem. If your eyebrows are extremely droopy, your doctor may advise correcting them first and following up with upper eyelid surgery several weeks later (see chapter 11). Sometimes it is easier to judge how much skin to remove from the upper eyelids after the eyebrows have been repositioned. Whether your doctor advises the forehead lift or the direct eyebrow lift, either type of surgery can raise your eyebrows and dramatically open the upper third of your face.

Wrinkles—Good and Bad

A forehead lift will not totally eliminate the lines on your forehead. Nor would you want it to.

Some forehead lines are caused by the natural movement of the muscles beneath the skin. They become more prominent when you scowl or raise your eyebrows. As a muscle tightens, it shortens, and the overlying skin is pulled into folds. "Your facial expressions can be very eloquent," explains a facial plastic surgeon from Omaha, Neb., "and you don't want to lose all of those lines."

A forehead lift does not stretch the skin tight enough to remove every line. Excess wrinkling of the forehead often can be improved with a chemical peel, which strengthens and thickens the upper layers of the skin, removing fine wrinkles and decreasing deeper wrinkles in the process (see chapter 16).

"We need our facial muscles and skin lines to help us communicate, but very deep lines on the forehead and between the eyebrows can communicate the wrong thing," the surgeon from Nebraska says. Eyebrow or forehead lifting combined with chemical peeling can reduce that scowling expression you see in the mirror but do not feel inside.

Forehead or eyebrow surgery also may be combined with a facelift (see chapter 8) or a procedure to correct drooping eyelids or remove bags under the eyes (see chapter 11).

15

Scars and Skin Problems

IT WAS A PERFECTLY FINE SPRING DAY, with no premonition of the disaster about to occur, when Doris P., a young Florida woman, was hurled off a motorcycle and skidded face down along the pavement. The impact cruelly tore the right side of her upper lip and her lower right eyelid.

Emergency surgery repaired the damage, but while healing the two scars contracted, pulling Doris' lip upward at an unpleasant angle and contorting the eyelid downward. "I looked gruesome," she admits.

Facial plastic surgery was able to change Doris' looks as well as her outlook. Her surgeon used a technique called a Z-plasty to release the contracted scars and reconstructed her lower eyelid using a flap of skin borrowed from the upper lid. "I look like a normal person again!" the young lady rejoices today.

Few things are more devastating to a person's self-image than an unsightly scar or blemish on the face. Whether it's a relatively small acne

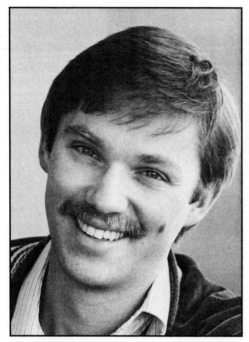 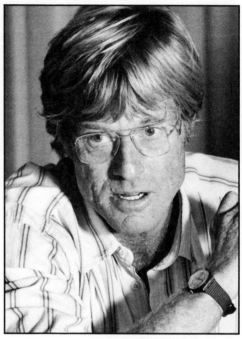

Facial skin imperfections do not always warrant correction. A rugged complexion certainly has not hurt Robert Redford's career, nor has Richard Thomas' mole thwarted his life on stage and screen.

scar or facial tumors that make others turn away in horror, facial irregularities cause immense emotional turmoil.

A large or unusual scar on the face can draw unwanted attention, making it difficult for other people to relate to you in a normal way. You may find it hard to be taken seriously in the professional world—and, of course, an ugly blemish can wreak havoc in your personal life. Some scars may even interfere with the normal functioning of your facial structures, such as your eyelid or lip.

Indeed, it is an unusual person who does not have several scars by adulthood. Most scars fade to near invisibility with time and do not cause a problem. But sometimes a scar—particularly one on the face—is impossible to hide. It may be unusually wide or long, or go across the natural creases and contours of the face. It may be raised above or sunken into the surrounding skin surface, or it may be a different color than the surrounding area.

Or perhaps your problem is not a scar but an unsightly mole, a large birthmark, or some other disfiguring facial blemish. If it interferes with your lifestyle or causes you undue anguish, facial plastic surgery may provide the answer.

What Is a Scar?

Scar tissue forms during the body's normal healing process. Scars occur when all of the layers of the skin are cut through. They can result from traumatic injury, burns, infections such as acne, and any type of surgery, including facial plastic surgery. Sometimes, particularly with men, a scar can lend a rakish air, an aura of manliness and mystery. Most often, though, they are just plain unattractive.

"Scarring cannot be prevented," explains a facial plastic surgeon from Vero Beach, Fla. "Nor do scars go away—once you have developed scar tissue, it will be there forever."

The news is not all bad, however. Careful planning and skillful surgical techniques can minimize the formation of noticeable scars. For instance, for individuals planning a facelift or other facial plastic surgery, the surgeon will plan the procedure so that scars fall in natural skin creases or the hairline, where they will be scarcely noticeable.

Three common types of scars can be improved by facial plastic surgery:

- *Hypertrophic or "overdeveloped" scars* are an excess of scar tissue that develops after an injury or surgical incision. This scar tissue appears redder in color and firmer in texture than the surrounding skin and is elevated from it.
- *Keloid scars* are similar to hypertrophic scars, but they continue to grow and enlarge with time, literally piling up scar tissue. The tendency to develop keloid scars may be genetic, as these scars tend to run in families. The areas most likely to develop keloid scars are the earlobes, chin, and neck.

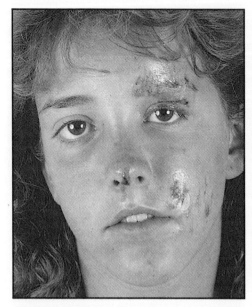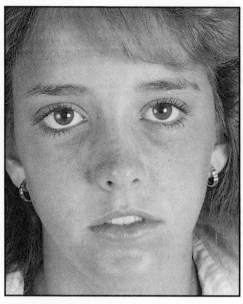

Surgery is not the only way to improve scars. Given sufficient time and proper care, scars may disappear by themselves, as occurred with this young woman. Mother Nature's ability to heal is one reason facial plastic surgeons often recommend waiting for six months or a year before seeking surgery to improve scars.

- *Acne scars* are the most common type of facial scarring and result from acne infections. This type is scarring usually is treated with dermabrasion (see chapter 16).

How Scar Revision Surgery Can Help

Scars cannot be erased or removed. Once the skin is cut all the way through, a scar will be there forever. Removal of a deep cancer, for instance, may leave a pit or depression. Emergency surgery to close open wounds after a serious accident may have to be done hurriedly, without regard for how the scars will ultimately look. And victims of thermal or chemical burns can suffer serious disfigurement despite the best medical care.

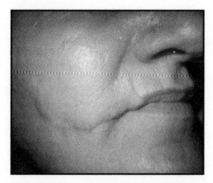 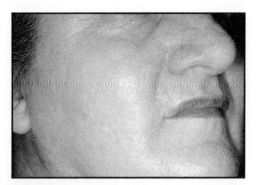

The lines of a straight scar can be broken up and thereby become less visible.

The goal of scar revision surgery, then, is to improve the appearance of an unsightly or disfiguring scar by trading it for one that is smaller and less conspicuous and, perhaps, easier to camouflage with makeup.

Facial plastic surgeons can excise a scar (remove it by cutting it out), making a smoother and neater scar, perhaps injecting steroids around the incision to reduce inflammation and prevent the formation of hypertrophic scars. They can break up long scars to make them more irregular and therefore less noticeable. They can relocate a scar so that it falls in a natural fold. And they can fill depressions and smooth raised surfaces of the skin.

No one can predict what the final appearance of a scar will be, especially since scars get worse before they get better. It takes at least six months and sometimes as long as two years for a scar to "mature" or reach the stage where no further change will occur. Incisions and injuries heal in stages. At first, tiny new blood vessels form in the area to help speed healing, causing the scar to look red and noticeable. As collagen fibers begin to be laid down, the new scar looks raised and lumpy. This may last for up to six weeks. Then the scar begins to shrink and soften—a process that may continue for a year or more.

The final appearance of a scar also depends on an individual's own ability to heal—some people have a tendency to scar more than others. Older people may heal with less scarring than the young. Children heal so well that they may actually "overheal," resulting in larger and more

Be Gone, Port Wine Stain

One of the most exciting uses of lasers in facial plastic surgery, according to a facial plastic surgeon from California, is in the treatment of port wine stains. These birthmarks tend to be very large and can be particularly disfiguring when they occur on the face. Until recently, they have been impossible to treat satisfactorily and their deep rosy hue—from whence comes their name—made them impervious to camouflage by makeup. Now laser technology makes it possible for some people with facial port wine stains to achieve an acceptable appearance using normal makeup.

The California surgeon likes to tell the heartwarming story of a girl who became a model after laser treatment of a large port wine stain on her face. A prisoner whose port wine stain had an adverse psychological effect underwent laser surgery and went on to a rehabilitation program. And a school teacher allergic to makeup quit teaching because of negative reaction from her students to her facial blemish. After treatment she was able to return to the classroom—without wearing makeup—with a totally acceptable appearance.

A particularly rewarding aspect of this new therapy, adds the surgeon from California, is that it seems safe for use on children. Scientists are proceeding cautiously at this time, but laser treatment has been used successfully to treat port wine stains on children under two years of age.

noticeable scars. It may take as long as 18 to 24 months for scars on young children to mature and as little as three months for scars on older persons. This is why surgeons frequently recommend waiting until a scar is fully mature before attempting scar revision surgery.

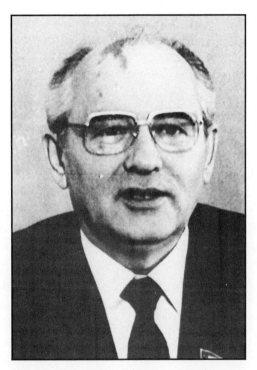

Probably the most well-known port wine stain in the world belongs to Mikhail Gorbachev.

Anyone unhappy about his or her appearance because of a facial scar can be considered a candidate for scar revision surgery. If the scar has fully matured and still looks objectionable, if the problem will not improve with time—a straight-line scar, or a J- or U-shaped scar, for instance—or if the scar is a hypertrophic or keloid type, the chances of improving its appearance through scar revision surgery are very good.

Although many months may go by before a scar can be revised, it is advisable for a surgical candidate to see a facial plastic surgeon soon after an accident so that the surgeon can observe the scar in its early healing stages, document how well the wound was put together, take photographs, and give the patient an idea of what can be done later.

Knowing that waiting is the right thing to do can be very reassuring to the patient.

The Techniques of Scar Revision

Estoria Moss suffered an automobile accident as a young woman that left her with a jagged scar running straight out from the side of her mouth. ''My jaw was cut in two places, and my lip was put back together crooked,'' she explains. For years she endured questions and sympathetic looks until she decided to see a facial plastic surgeon.

''A scar that is a straight line is very noticeable because it cuts across the natural folds of the face,'' says the surgeon from Florida. To correct this type of problem, the surgeon uses a technique called a ''geometric broken line closure.'' ''The goal,'' he explains, ''is to make the scar irregular, breaking it up so that it doesn't catch the eye quite as much. Instead of a straight line, the scar forms a tiny geometric pattern of little triangles or squares that meet each other. The result is a scar that blends in with the natural skin texture and is much less noticeable.''

''Knowing I look better really gave me a lift,'' says Moss. ''Facial plastic surgery really made a difference in my life.''

Z-plasty, the procedure used on both Moss and on Doris, the motorcycle accident victim, is designed to release a contracted scar. The surgeon makes an incision along the scar, then makes two little cuts above and below it at angles to form a Z. The two small flaps of skin are readjusted and carefully stitched, resulting in a smooth, narrow scar that does not pull the skin.

A similar technique is the running W-plasty, which breaks up a straight-line scar with an up-and-down pattern. More extensive reconstructive techniques also are possible. Using a procedure called serial excision, facial plastic surgeons can remove a large scar a little at a time over a period of months. After each procedure, the remaining skin is stretched and the incision closed. After this heals, a little more of the scar is removed, until all that remains is a narrow line.

Yet another technique makes use of multiple flaps of healthy skin that are loosened at one end and repositioned to cover damaged areas.

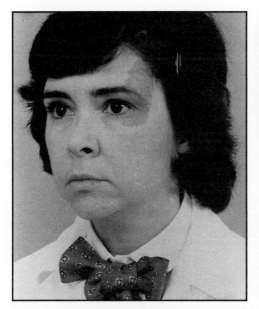 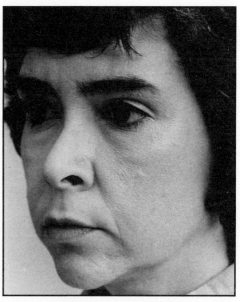

Lasers actually vaporize port wine stains. They can remove tatoos, too.

This procedure is especially useful for treating burn victims and others who have suffered extensive injuries.

Lasers Help Eliminate Skin Blemishes

One of the newest and most amazing advances in facial plastic surgery has been the use of the laser, truly a state-of-the-art development.

"Laser technology has many applications in facial plastic surgery," says a facial plastic surgeon from Santa Barbara, Calif., "particularly in the treatment of skin blemishes." Lasers as a surgical tool offer better precision, less bleeding, and less pain; they seem to seal off nerve endings as well as blood vessels instantly as they cut through the skin.

Three kinds of laser equipment are currently being used by facial plastic surgeons. All three types of lasers use light from that section of the electromagnetic spectrum between ultraviolet and infrared rays. How each affects tissue depends on the wavelength, the power density of the

Blemishes or Birthmarks?
There Is Hope

The same surgical techniques for revising facial scars also can help individuals with unsightly blemishes or birthmarks. The following skin problems can be treated through facial plastic surgery.

- Colored birthmarks, such as strawberry marks or ''port wine stains''
- Dark, hairy birthmarks, which have some potential for becoming malignant
- Noncancerous moles that are unattractive or slowly enlarging
- Small cysts, which may enlarge slowly or become infected
- Oversized freckles, or lentigines, sometimes called ''liver spots''
- Spider veins, or telangiectases—threadlike vessels just beneath the skin surface that usually appear on the cheeks or nose
- Rosacea—small, firm, reddish bumps on the face, generally occurring in middle age
- Rhinophyma, a severe rosacea with enlarged oil glands that leads to a gradual thickening of the nasal skin, actually enlarging the nose (the W. C. Fields look)
- Warty thickenings or growths known as seborrheic keratoses, which often appear after age 45 or 50
- Rough, reddish patches called actinic keratoses, caused by prolonged exposure to the sun and most common in fair-skinned people
- Small, elevated, yellowish plaques called xanthelasma, generally occurring on the eyelids
- Multiple raised, brownish bumps on the upper cheeks near the eyes, known as dermatosis papulosa nigra and occurring most often in orientals and blacks

- Skin-colored bumps called syringomas, which occur on or near the lower eyelids or along the side of the nose
- Small, slightly raised white bumps called milia, which occur most frequently on women's faces and resemble pimples but have no central pore
- Ear keloids, which may follow an injury or ear piercing
- Skin tags, which may form on the lower neck or armpits, most common in overweight people

beam, and the type of tissue. Basically, in laser surgery, light is shot through a tube that contains one of three types of gas: CO_2, argon, or YAG (yetrium aluminum gamet). Stimulated either by direct current or radio frequency, the excited photons begin to bounce or resonate between fully or partially reflective mirrors situated at either end of the tube. The fully amplified light or laser beam is let out through a shutter at one end of the tube.

Depending on the type of gas used, the beam vaporizes or excises the tissue. Tissue vaporizes as the CO_2 beam absorbs water. The YAG laser causes more coagulation than vaporization. The argon laser, which produces a blue-green light visible to the naked eye, is absorbed by red tissues, not water.

A procedure called laser-brasion has been used to peel off successive layers of warts and hyperkeratoses, and photodynamic therapy, an experimental treatment that involves injecting a drug that localizes within the tumor, has shown some exciting possibilities.

Spider veins, "red nose," and similar blemishes can be treated with a laser device that has a needle-nose probe. The surgeon places the needle directly into the vein and actually "spot welds" the individual vessels. The sudden coagulation minimizes the damage to the vessel and has proven to be a highly effective form of treatment. One caveat: Since laser technology is new, make certain that the facial plastic surgeon you select has had a reasonable amount of hands-on experience.

A Face You Can Live With

For those with an unfortunate facial scar or disfiguring blemish, chances are good that modern facial plastic surgery techniques can help correct the problem and minimize disfigurement so that it can be successfully camouflaged with cosmetics.

Few complications or risks are associated with scar revision surgery. Often the procedure can be done in a facial plastic surgeon's office or an outpatient surgical facility. Costs for this type of surgery vary widely depending on the extent and complexity of the defect. Sometimes two or three procedures are necessary to correct the problem. Insurance may cover the cost of the treatment, so you should consult a representative of your insurance company in advance.

Whatever your problem, facial plastic surgery may help give you a face you will be glad to see in the mirror—and thus a new outlook on life.

16

Blemishes, Wrinkles, and Sun-damaged Skin

SINCE THE DAYS OF ANTIQUITY, women have desired a smooth, clear complexion. Peaches and cream complexion, skin like milk and honey: Unblemished skin always has been associated with beauty.

In an earlier age, women went to great lengths to keep their skin protected with parasols and sunbonnets. Today's more active woman is not willing to give up sunbathing, skiing, gardening, jogging, tennis, cycling, and a 101 other reasons for being out in the sun. Skin that has been abused by the sun ages more quickly—especially for those with thinner "Anglo-Saxon" complexions (see chapter 3)—often leading to premature wrinkling and the formation of leathery skin. Men are used to a coarser complexion, but they, too, are not happy when the outdoor life gives them wrinkled eyes and a tired appearance.

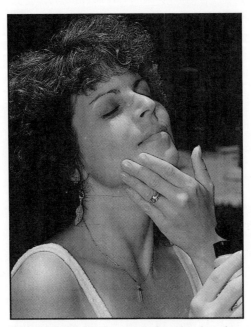

Protecting the skin from sun abuse has long been a priority of women who desire a clear, lovely complexion.

It is Not Just the Sun's Fault

But what about those who protect themselves from the sun? The ravages of time still will leave their mark—in the form of lines, wrinkles, and surface irregularities.

Everyone experiences wrinkling as they get older. Some people (see chapters 2 and 3) wrinkle more than others. If you look older than your age because of a network of lines and wrinkles around your eyes, above your upper lip, or all over your face, chemical peeling may help you regain your youthful glow. It can take years of sun damage off your face—and keep it off unless the sun abuse continues.

"Every surgeon has a favorite way of taking care of problems," says a facial plastic surgeon from Birmingham, Ala., "and it is often possible to accomplish the same result with different methods. But in general, chemical peeling is used primarily for wrinkles, and dermabrasion is used

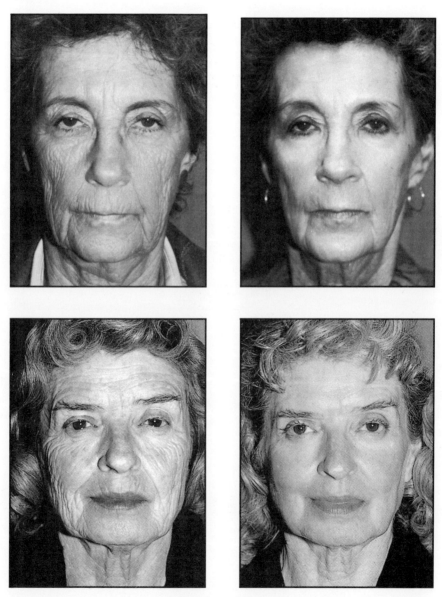

The full face chemical peel offers an excellent way to eliminate wrinkles. Many women, like the two pictured above, consider it an alternative to a facelift.

primarily for scars." Both chemical peeling and dermabrasion remove the damaged top layers of the skin so that new skin can grow in its place.

"I tell my patients that chemical peeling is like putting turpentine on an old table covered with multiple coats of paint," says the surgeon from Alabama. "The chemical causes the old paint to blister and come off, revealing a fresh, clean surface beneath. On the other hand, dermabrasion is like sanding a scratch on the surface of a wooden table—the old surface is removed, and the scratch disappears."

A third method of improving the contours of the face—the use of injectable fillers—gives facial plastic surgeons yet another weapon to use in the fight against visible signs of aging.

Chemical Peel Unveils New Skin

"It's just an incredible process, worth every penny of it," says Patti Lieber, who liked her facial plastic surgery results so much that she has had several facial procedures. "First I had an eyelid tuck, and then I had chemical peeling done around my eyes and on my forehead," she explains. "It worked beautifully. Then I had a facelift, followed by a full-face chemical peel.

"I do some modeling and I'm a professional singer, so I'm constantly in the public eye. People don't believe I have five boys, all in college. They're so proud of the way I look now. My youngest tells me, 'Mom, you look so young!'"

Is a Chemical Peel For You?

Chemical face peeling is not a substitute for a facelift. Individuals with loose skin need surgery to remove the excess skin, but a facelift does not remove fine lines and wrinkles. For this, you need chemical peeling, a procedure that removes the top layer of lined skin to reveal new, glowing, unwrinkled skin beneath.

Chemical peeling frequently is done after a facelift (chapter 8) or eyelid surgery (chapter 11), as in Lieber's case, to remove the fine wrinkles that remain. "Imagine a dress or suit that is too large and ill-fit-

The Science of a Chemical Peel

The skin has two main layers: the "epidermis" and the "dermis." The deeper layer—the dermis—is composed mainly of collagen fibers. Under a microscope, these fibers look like spaghetti thrown on a table—long, thin strands with no organized pattern. The dermis is divided into two layers: the "papillary dermis" on top and the deeper "reticular dermis."

If a cut or injury penetrates into only the papillary dermis, you will heal without a scar. However, if the injury goes deeper—into the reticular dermis—a scar results. The chemical peel removes the epidermis and penetrates only into the papillary dermis. As the skin heals, the epidermis is rejuvenated and the collagen fibers of the dermis become shorter, thicker, and more organized, which tightens the skin. This process takes about nine to 12 months, so final results may not be apparent until about one year after the procedure is done.

ting after you have lost a lot of weight," says a facial plastic surgeon from Indianapolis, Ind. "A good tailor might perform alterations to remove the excess fabric and make the garment fit properly. But alterations alone will not remove the fine wrinkles; to finish the job, the tailor still needs to steam the garment." In the same way, he explains, the facial plastic surgeon may remove excess skin with facelift surgery, but a chemical peel still may be needed to rejuvenate the skin and eliminate facial wrinkling.

If the procedure is done in conjunction with other facial plastic surgery, you may be advised to wait several weeks or months after the surgery before undergoing chemical face peeling, to allow the skin tissues to heal properly.

Chemical peeling also may be done alone. "I wasn't interested in a facelift, just in getting rid of all the little lines on my face," says Toni D.

"Chemical peeling made such a difference. I feel better about myself now. It's a good feeling."

Chemical peels may be used on the entire face or in specific areas where excess wrinkling is a problem. Your facial plastic surgeon will advise you whether you need a full-face peel or treatment in a smaller area. A chemical peel in the area around the mouth is called a "perioral peel"; a peel in the area around the eyes is called a "periorbital peel."

Types of Chemical Peels

Three basic types of chemical peels are used on the face. They include:

- *Salicylic acid peels.* Salicylic acid is a very mild chemical used for facial peels. This type of peel may be performed by a cosmetologist. The results of this treatment are temporary.
- *Trichloroacetic acid (TCA) peels.* This type of peel must be performed by a physician. Trichloroacetic acid comes in varying strengths—the more concentrated the solution, the more deeply it penetrates facial tissues. TCA peels provide longer-lasting results than salicylic acid peels, but they are not as long-lasting as phenol peels. TCA peels are easily performed in the doctor's office, however, and the healing time is considerably shorter than that required following a phenol peel.
- *Phenol peels.* Facial plastic surgeons perform this type of chemical face peel most often. The results of a phenol peel can be dramatic and can last for years. If you have deep facial wrinkles or if your skin has a weathered, leathery texture, a phenol chemical peel may be the best choice for you. A phenol peel takes several weeks to heal, though you probably will be able to apply makeup over the treated area after about two weeks.

Painting the Face

Before the chemical peel begins, the facial plastic surgeon will have you remove all makeup and wash your face several times with an an-

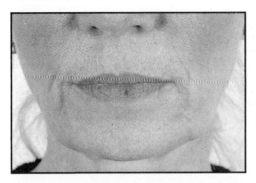 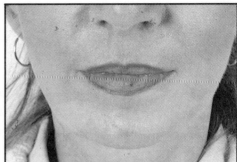

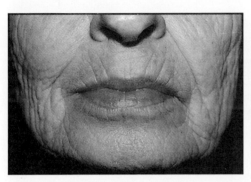 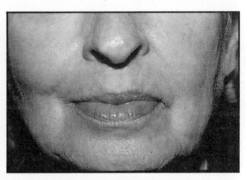

The younger woman (at top) had both a facelift and a chemical peel around her mouth. The older woman had only a chemical peel. The peel smooths the skin around the mouth and reduces laugh lines and the vertical wrinkles next to the lips.

tibiotic soap. Then your skin will be cleansed thoroughly with substances that further remove deep facial oils. This will allow the chemical solution to penetrate your skin properly.

The chemical solution is skillfully applied with a cotton-tipped applicator to specific areas in a sequential pattern. You will notice a burning sensation as the solution is applied, which stops after about 10 to 15 seconds. Twenty to 30 minutes later, you will begin to feel a mild burning sensation similar to that of a sunburn. This will continue for the next four to six hours, but you should feel no further pain or discomfort after that. Your surgeon will give you a mild pain reliever if you need it to minimize or eliminate this minor discomfort. How uncomfortable is it? ''It felt like getting a burn on the stove,'' recalls Patti Lieber, ''but it only hurt for a few minutes. There is definitely some pain, but the results are worth the little bit of suffering.''

For small areas such as around the eyes or mouth, no sedation is required. But for a full-face peel, your surgeon may recommend ''twilight'' anesthesia, a mild sedation similar to that used for dental work. A sedative is administered intravenously, and cardiac and blood pressure monitors are used.

After the chemical peel is completed, a dressing is applied to protect the surface and keep it moist. Different dressings are used, depending on the preference of the surgeon—some like antibiotic ointments or moisturizing creams, others apply a bland vegetable shortening, and still others use gauze dressings or tape that is applied to the face and removed after several days.

Patients who have had this procedure recommend not being alone the first night. ''It helps to have someone with you who really cares about you,'' advises Toni D. ''The pain was not that much since I was sedated and pretty much out of it. It was more traumatic for my daughter, who stayed with me and kept ointment on my face constantly.''

The First Few Days Are the Worst

Considerable swelling and crusting will occur, and many patients have difficulty realizing in advance how bad they will look temporarily. ''I tell my patients to think of the worst thing they have ever seen, multiply it times 10, and they are still not even close to how horrible they will look during the first two weeks after a chemical peel,'' says the facial plastic surgeon from Indiana. Adds Patti Lieber, ''You look like an orangutan!''

Frequent showering often is advised to help moisten facial ''crusts'' and ''float'' them away. ''This technique facilitates the healing process,'' says the surgeon from Indiana, ''and greatly reduces or eliminates discomfort during the healing process.''

''I worked very hard at doing exactly what the doctor told me to do,'' says Toni D. ''I sprayed my face for 15 minutes every two hours for the

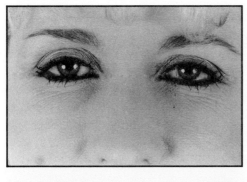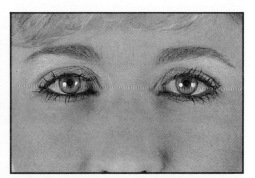

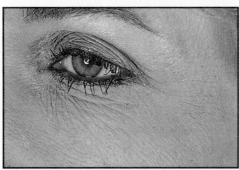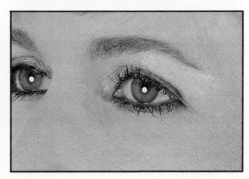

When a chemical peel is performed on the upper and lower eyelids and on the region between the eyebrows, there is a decrease in the fine wrinkles in those areas.

first week, and the redness left very quickly. I believe good care afterwards had a lot to do with that.''

It takes about 14 days after peeling for the skin to ''resurface.'' The new skin is delicate, pink, and free of wrinkles. You may feel that your skin has tightened as well. Although not all wrinkles can be removed, you should notice a significant improvement.

Your skin will be very red for weeks following a chemical peel, but this can be camouflaged quite well with makeup. The redness fades gradually over six to eight weeks, and most people regain their normal skin tone.

Frequently Asked Questions
About Chemical Peels

Will my chemical face peel need to be repeated?

Usually not. Phenol peels generally are very long-lasting. Occasionally, however, some areas may need to be touched up.

Who is not a good candidate for a chemical peel?

If you have a very dark complexion, you may not be a good candidate for a chemical peel because of the lightening effect that may take place. In addition, anyone who has a decreased ability for the skin to regenerate should not have a chemical peel. This might include those who have had x-ray treatments to their face for acne, those who have taken certain drugs, and individuals with burn scars. These conditions may significantly reduce the ability of your skin to regenerate. Also, persons who have serious heart or kidney disorders may not be appropriate candidates for the treatment because of the way that the chemical is passed out of the body. Your facial plastic surgeon can help you decide if chemical peeling is right for you.

Are wrinkles the only reason to have a chemical face peel?

Chemical face peels can be used to remove precancerous lesions on the skin caused by excess exposure to the sun. Another use: Some women develop a condition called melasma, also known as "the mask of pregnancy." Phenol chemical peels can remove such abnormal areas of dark pigmentation.

Will a chemical peel remove the dark circles under my eyes?

Bagginess under the eyes usually is the result of excess fatty tissue, and the resulting bulge can cast a shadow that appears as a darkness under the eyes. If you have this problem, a procedure called blepharoplasty—eyelid surgery—would be the appropriate treatment (see chapter 11). Some people, however, have extra pigment in the eyelid area. If this is the case, a chemical peel may help you.

Will a chemical peel eliminate the large pores on my face?

No, chemical peeling does not affect pore size; pores are the openings of oil glands.

Will a chemical peel help to reduce my acne scars?

It depends on how deep your scars are. Often a chemical peel does not significantly improve acne scars, but there may be a benefit in some cases. Dermabrasion generally is recommended for acne scars. Your facial plastic surgeon can advise you after a thorough examination.

Is much pain associated with a chemical peel?

A slight burning sensation when the solution is applied, lasting 10-15 seconds, and four to six hours of a burning sensation similar to a mild sunburn following the procedure should be all the discomfort experienced. Pain medications are prescribed to make the patient comfortable during this time.

Complexion Changes Are Possible

Some people, however, end up with complexions that are a bit lighter than before the peel; and a few experience considerable lightening of their skin, which requires the use of makeup all the time to camouflage the peeled areas. This is important to know—if you never wear makeup, you probably should not consider having a phenol chemical peel. Also, individuals with dark complexions often are advised not to have such a peel.

Why does chemical peeling sometimes lighten the skin? Two factors determine the color of your complexion—the thickness of the epidermis and the amount of melanin (pigment) in your skin. After a chemical peel,

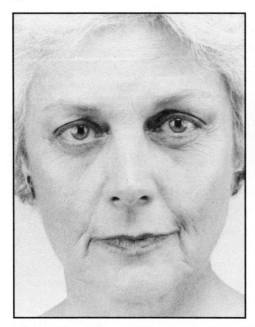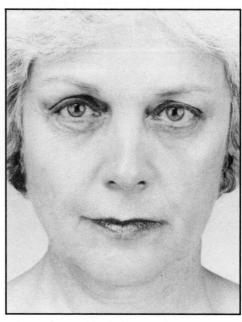

Filling deep wrinkles with an injectable material like collagen is a relatively new treatment method.

the new epidermis may be a different thickness than before. Another possibility is that the phenol used may break down some of the melanin in the pigment cells.

Postoperative Care is Important

Patients who have had a chemical peel must avoid exposure to the sun for several months. Tanning during the first six months after a chemical peel can affect pigmentation and cause a splotchy appearance. When normal outdoor activities are resumed, a sun screen (SPF 15 or higher) is recommended on the recently peeled areas.

If your facial skin is lined or wrinkled but not too saggy, you might be thrilled with the difference chemical peeling can make. "My family loved me before," says Toni, "but they are proud that I look so much better now. Recently my granddaughter said, 'You're beginning to look like a teenager, Granny!'"

"I get quite a few comments," adds Lieber. "I think it's worth the satisfaction. I get a great lift from people saying, 'Oh, you look so young, Patti, what have you done with yourself?' I think it's super, and I'm all for it."

Dermabrasion—A Facial Sanding Alternative

During dermabrasion, the surgeon uses a rotating brush to "sand" off the top layers of the skin. Sometimes dermabrasion is used to treat severe cases of cystic acne that have failed to respond to other medical treatment. "It's the ultimate procedure for cleansing the skin," the facial plastic surgeon from Alabama explains. "Although it certainly should not be used for every case of acne, dermabrasion can help in some cases that don't improve with conventional treatment."

Dermabrasion also is used to remove old acne scars, birthmarks and other large areas of excess pigmentation, and raised scar tissue. "Some of the problems treated by dermabrasion also may respond to chemical peeling, laser surgery, or other techniques," says the surgeon from Alabama. "It is up to the surgeon to choose the procedure he or she feels most comfortable with and that is likely to yield the best results. Sometimes a combination of procedures is the best choice."

Local anesthetics and topical freezing agents render dermabrasion relatively painless. Mild intravenous anesthesia is used when large areas of the face are treated. The procedure usually is done in the surgeon's office or in an outpatient surgical facility.

Immediately after dermabrasion, the treated area looks like a skinned knee, and a yellowish fluid oozes from it. This is part of the normal healing process, and it begins to subside after 24 hours. Some patients experience throbbing or stinging, which is controlled with a mild nonaspirin pain reliever and ice compresses. Swelling, ranging from moderate to severe, usually is worst on the second or third day after dermabrasion and then begins to subside.

Healing after dermabrasion is similar to healing after a chemical peel. The area is bathed gently several times each day to keep the crusts soft, and an ointment or dressing is applied daily. The crusts fall off about 10

Whence Cometh Wrinkles

A number of factors contribute to excessive and early wrinkling, explains a facial plastic surgeon from Indianapolis, Ind. These include:

- Exposure to the sun. Those who work outdoors, participate frequently in outdoor recreational activities, or spend long hours suntanning on the beach are at increased risk of wrinkling prematurely.
- Exposure to the wind. Like the sun, wind dries the skin, causing it to age prematurely. Think of the typical picture of an old sailor or fisherman who has spent his life battling the elements—his face is brown and leathery, deeply etched with wrinkles.
- Cigarette smoking. If you smoke, particularly if you started at an early age, your facial skin may be more wrinkled than that of someone the same age who never smoked.
- Poor-fitting dentures. A dental appliance that does not fit properly may strain the tissues around the mouth, causing small lines and wrinkles.

to 14 days after surgery, and the new skin appears intensely pink and fades to normal color over a period of weeks. Makeup can be applied after the area heals, and excess sun must be avoided to prevent blotchiness.

Injectable Fillers—Plumping the Skin

Not all facial plastic surgery procedures involve cutting and redraping the skin. It is sometimes possible to inject special "filler" materials to improve the contours of the face. Some problems that may respond well to injectable fillers:

- a change in the contours of the face caused by accident or disease;
- acne scarring that is not excessively deep;
- congenital facial depressions, such as underdeveloped cheek-bones;
- depressions caused by the breakdown of fat pads in the face which occurs naturally with age; and
- deep scars or wrinkles.

Injectable fillers also are used occasionally to enhance the results of other facial procedures, such as rhinoplasty.

Injectable fillers include plastic materials, collagen, and certain fats. The filler is injected into the skin with very fine needles. The material fills out the depression, raising it and thus making it less noticeable. The major drawback is the procedure's lack of permanence. Most injectable fillers are absorbed by the body in time; thus, the procedure must be repeated every nine months to two years for optimum results.

Collagen is a gel-like substance that is similar to the structural protein of the skin and other body tissues. It often is referred to by the brand names of Zyplast and Zyderm. Injectable collagen is a highly purified form derived from animal tissues. Complications are rare, but collagen has been known to cause allergic reactions in some patients.

Many women have regular collagen injections to smooth out the crevices that form in the area just above the upper lip. Men tend to seek the treatment for deep frown lines. Since the procedure often does not require anesthesia, it is possible to have the injections done and then to return directly to work. Your facial plastic surgeon will freeze the area of the skin to be injected; however, there is a burning sensation from the needle, especially in the tender lip area.

An even newer technique—lipoinjection—entails extracting the fat from another part of the patient's own body, often the thigh or abdomen area, and using it as the filler material. Like collagen, however, lipoinjection is temporary. The advantage of both these procedures is cost effectiveness: In some cases, injections cost less than a chemical peel and may be the best solution for an individual whose wrinkles are not severe.

Can Skin Creams Treat Aging?

Much excitement has been generated over Retin-A, a cream derived from vitamin A that primarily has been used to treat facial acne. Some long term users began noticing a decrease in facial wrinkles, and a small-scale study at the University of Michigan presented strong evidence that topical applications of Retin-A over a four-month period do improve the skin surface.

Since the cream penetrates only the top layer of the skin—the epidermis—the most impressive improvement occurs in fine wrinkling, a relatively early sign of aging. The improvement is somewhat subtle, and those with severely damaged skin benefit much less, regardless of the length of treatment.

Retin-A does not have the same effects as the more concentrated TCA peels or phenol chemical face peels. Moreover, a number of unpleasant side effects have been noted in long term users, primarily dermatitis (inflamation of the skin). Retin-A must be prescribed by a physician, and patients should carefully follow their doctors' advice about its proper usage.

Retin-A is no substitute for a chemical peel or other forms of facial plastic surgery. Information is not yet available as to what happens to skin when the drug is discontinued and possible dangerous side effects with prolonged use. If you are considering using Retin-A, find out as much as possible about it in advance, and approach its use with extreme caution.

The results of injectable fillers can be dramatic, according to a facial plastic surgeon from Westport, Conn. "I had one patient, a psychiatrist, whose sunken cheeks greatly affected her personality. She would never look up at me. After the fat injection, she underwent a complete personality change. She became very happy with herself."

Which form of injectable filler is best for you? This is a question best answered by your surgeon. The answer depends on the nature of your problem and the doctor's preferences and experience. Properly used, injectable fillers can help smooth your facial contour; eliminate some scars or deep wrinkles; delay the need for a facelift; or complement a facelift (chapter 8), rhinoplasty (chapter 9), or other surgical procedure.

17

Liposuction of the Face and Neck

"NO MATTER HOW MUCH I diet or exercise, I just cannot get rid of my double chin!"

This is a common problem for both women and men, and until recently, not much could be done to resolve it. That has now changed with the advent of a revolutionary new surgical technique called liposuction.

Liposuction (also called suction-assisted lipectomy) is a method for removing small pockets of excess fat cells from certain parts of the body through a tiny incision. The technique provides facial plastic surgeons with the opportunity to sculpt the face and neck in ways that were just not possible before.

Consider John H., a 38-year-old dentist who has always hated his weak, double chin. He had two consultations with a facial plastic surgeon who showed him the changes that were possible on a computer imaging screen. John liked what he saw and chose to have liposuction of the neck and a chin implant (see chapter 12). He had surgery on a Thursday afternoon and returned to work Monday morning.

"Finally, I have a well-defined chin and neckline," he says with exuberance. "And no one even knows I had the operation. My dental staff have all said I look better and younger, but they couldn't say why."

Lipo What?

Liposuction is relatively new as a facial plastic surgery procedure. It was developed in Europe nearly 20 years ago and introduced in the United States in the early 1980s. American surgeons, many of them members of the American Academy of Facial Plastic and Reconstructive Surgery, further refined and perfected the technique, developing both new instruments and improved techniques. Today liposuction is known as a safe and effective procedure that is helping millions of people achieve the look they want.

Who gets liposuction? Lots of people, facial plastic surgeons report. The use of liposuction in the United States has grown tremendously in the past 10 years with more than 100,000 men and women having the procedure done each year. But misconceptions abound as to what liposuction can accomplish.

"Liposuction is definitely not a substitute for weight loss and exercise in overweight individuals," warns a facial plastic surgeon from Cincinnati, Ohio. "If excessive facial fat is part of an overall weight problem, surgery will provide only a temporary solution."

Fat cells, he says, increase and decrease in size, not in number. Liposuction, therefore, is helpful when abnormal numbers of fat cells are present in isolated areas. It is beneficial for persons who have specific problems, like the dentist, John H., or Cindy Y., a 25-year-old executive secretary who exercises regularly and maintains a normal weight. Yet, she told the surgeon in exasperation, "I have always had this round face. It makes me look fat when I'm not, and what is worse is that I have a weak chin with a bulge beneath. I'm too young to have a double chin."

Cindy decided on facial and neck liposuction along with a chin implant. The procedure was done under twilight anesthesia, in which mild

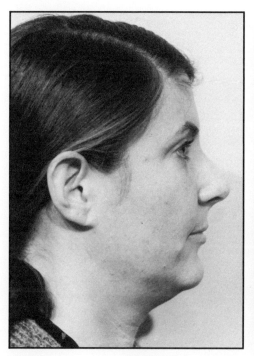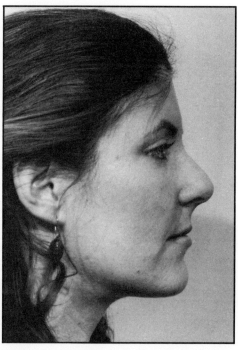

Liposuction can give a dramatically new look to the face, as these before (at left) and after photos demonstrate.

sedatives are given orally and intravenously and combined with local anesthesia, inducing "twilight sleep" and rendering the procedure painless. Cindy returned to work after five days. "I had absolutely no pain except for some minor chin discomfort," she recalls. "I didn't think I would ever have a smooth neckline and a chin—this is exactly what I wanted."

For some individuals, liposuction must be performed with a facelift (see chapter 8) to obtain the best results. The reason is that in younger persons, the skin is fairly elastic. After the excess fat is removed, the overlying skin collapses and shrinks. But with older patients, the elasticity of the skin often is poor, or there may be excessive skin that hangs loosely. If this is the case, a facelift or necklift can eliminate the sagging skin while liposuction takes care of the excess fat. This is analogous to taking the slack from one's clothes with alterations following substantial weight loss.

Before the advent of liposuction, excessive fat in the cheek, jowl, or neck areas of a patient undergoing a facelift or necklift had to be removed by cutting it out. This method often left undesirable irregularities, particularly under the chin. The liposuction technique, on the other hand, generally eliminates such deformities and yields a smooth, well-sculpted appearance.

How the Surgery Works

The facial plastic surgeon will evaluate your face and neck carefully during your first consultation to determine whether you are a candidate for lipsuction alone, liposuction combined with a chin implant, or liposuction combined with a facelift.

Liposuction usually is done in an office-based surgical suite or an outpatient surgery center. Rarely is it necessary to spend a night in the hospital. Nor is it necessary to undergo general anesthesia. With the use of twilight anesthesia, you probably will sleep through the procedure.

The incisions made during liposuction are tiny. Your surgeon may make an incision under your chin in a natural crease or in the natural fold under each earlobe. Scars are almost never visible once they are completely healed. The suction instrument, known as a cannula, is inserted through the incision, into the area with excess fat (along the jawline, in the cheeks, or under the chin in the neck). The fat is removed by ''vacuuming.''

The surgeon determines how much fat to remove by feeling the skin and pinching the tissues. If a chin implant is to be placed at the same time to correct a receding chin, it can be inserted through the same small incision. When a facelift is necessary, the incisions are simply extended from the earlobe in an upward direction in front of and behind the ears.

Is Liposuction Right for You?

Are you a candidate for liposuction? Here, from a facial plastic surgeon from Cincinnati, Ohio, are some questions that may help you decide:

- Are you young and not particularly overweight but unhappy because of a round face that appears fat? If you would like more of a classic oval face, and to perhaps bring your cheekbones and chin out of hiding, you might benefit from liposuction of the cheeks, jowls, and neck.

- Do your double chin and neck seem to run together, so that people can hardly tell where your face ends and your neck begins? Liposuction with the insertion of a chin implant (see chapter 12) can strengthen your profile without dramatically altering your appearance.

- Are double chins a family trait? If you have a hereditary tendency to accumulate fat under your chin and jowls but you have good skin elasticity and feel too young for a facelift, you might be pleased to see the difference simple liposuction of the area under your chin can make.

- Do you have not only excessive fat but loose skin that produces deep smile lines, saggy jowls, and a baggy neck? A facelift (see chapter 8) with liposuction done at the same time may be what is needed to restore your face to a natural, more youthful appearance.

Recovering from Liposuction

After the operation, a snug dressing is placed around your face and neck, and you may rest in the surgical facility for a short period before being driven home. The dressing is removed in the surgeon's office the

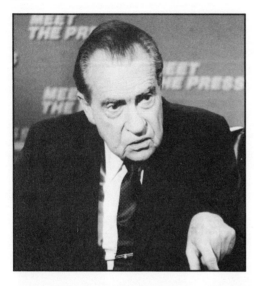

Celebrity offers no immunity to jowls, which plague many men and women as they grow older. Liposuction is often recommended to improve the condition.

next day, and you may be advised to wear a "chin strap"—an elastic bandage placed under the chin and tied on top of the head—for a few days and for several weeks at night.

Very little pain is associated with liposuction. Most patients experience some discomfort the first night, but after the dressing is removed most of the discomfort is ended, and the patient can function quite well at home. A regular diet can be resumed the next day unless a chin implant is involved. If so, chewing must be avoided for a week. Patients usually return to work within three to five days after liposuction; exercise, sports, and other strenuous activities can be resumed in seven to 10 days. When a facelift or other procedure has been done at the same time, the recovery time is slightly longer, but most people can return to work in 10 to 14 days.

Liposuction alone rarely causes bruising, but if a small amount of bruising does develop, makeup can be used immediately to cover it up. Improvement is noticeable immediately, but it may take three to six months to see the final results, after swelling diminishes completely and the skin returns to normal.

Complications and risks of liposuction in the face and neck are quite rare, the facial plastic surgeon from Ohio emphasizes. Occasionally, a patient may develop a slight hardness in the treated area—this is not visible and disappears in a few weeks. Slight irregularities usually smooth out during the healing period. It is extremely rare to have injuries to surrounding nerves and blood vessels. In fact, surgeons consider liposuction an exceedingly safe procedure.

The cost of facial liposuction varies from about $500 to $1,500, depending on which part of the face and neck is treated. These figures do not include fees for facial implants, a facelift, or other procedures done at the same time. There may be additional fees for the use of the surgical facility and the anesthetist. It is usually more economical to have the surgery performed in an office-based surgical center than in a hospital.

A Quick, Easy Way to a New, Trimmer You

Virginia P., a 56-year-old homemaker, has been healthy all her life and generally feels vivacious and socially active. She has always had a slight double chin, but in the past five years she has been dismayed by increasing sagging of her cheeks, jowls, and neck. Virginia wanted a rejuvenated look, and her facial plastic surgeon recommended both liposuction and a facelift.

The surgery was performed in an outpatient surgical facility, and, on the 11th day after surgery, Virginia attended an important social function with her husband, looking younger and feeling much more self-confident. "The best part," she says, "is that people comment about how good I look, but they have no idea that I've had facial surgery."

If, like Virginia, your face doesn't match your figure or your image of yourself, or if you are tired of putting up with a double chin, chubby cheeks, or other areas of localized facial fat that dieting and exercise won't touch, facial liposuction may be for you.

18

Hair Replacement

BALDNESS IS NOTHING NEW. Centuries ago, when Julius Caesar was courting Cleopatra, he combed his hair carefully to the side to cover the bald spot on top. Nor have the passing years made the condition any more palatable.

"Baldness is to men what wrinkles are to women," comments a facial plastic surgeon from Beverly Hills, Calif.

If you are male and over 30, chances are you have looked in the mirror and bemoaned the thinning of your hairline. The sad fact is that most men experience hair loss as they age. The lucky ones will only notice a little thinning around the temples or perhaps a receding hairline. But for many, growing older will mean growing balder—anything from a small bare spot at the crown to extensive hair loss over the front and top of the head. Doctors call this "male pattern baldness," and, if it's the story of your life, know that you are not alone. Most men begin to lose their hair as they reach their early 30s, and two-thirds of all men eventually are affected.

David R., a Wall Street executive with a worldwide financial services organization, is one of those who started losing his hair early. "My ap-

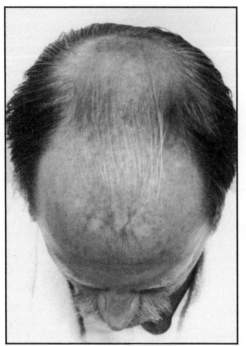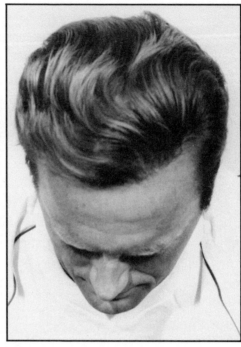

Flap surgery can produce gratifying results for balding men.

pearance is very important to me,'' he says, ''and I just wasn't ready to accept baldness. I was really unhappy, and I became very determined to find an answer.''

The answer, for David, was a revolutionary new procedure called scalp flap surgery. ''Now I have the hairline of a 16-year-old that will never be subject to male pattern baldness. I look great, and I love it,'' he reports.

Facial plastic surgery offers several alternatives to balding that are highly effective and permanent. Depending on the extent of your baldness and how your remaining hair is distributed, one of these options may be right for you.

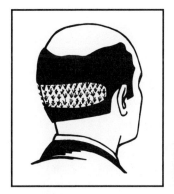 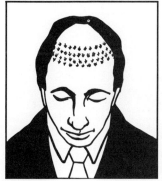 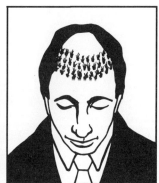

Figure A   *Figure B*   *Figure C*

Punch Graft Transplantation

Punch grafts—the "hair transplants" everyone has heard about—are the oldest method of hair replacement surgery and still the most common. The punch graft technique involves removing small, circular pieces of hair-bearing skin (about 1/6 inch in diameter) from the back of the head (figure A) and transplanting them to the top of the head, eliminating a small piece of bald skin. Usually 25 to 100 grafts are done at one time, depending on the size of the bald area (figure B).

Punch grafts can be done in a surgeon's office under local anesthesia. A bandage is left on overnight, and after a day or two you can wash your hair. You can resume most normal activities immediately after surgery, although you will have to avoid strenuous exercise and sweating. The stitches are removed 10 days after surgery.

Within six weeks the transplanted hair falls out, but, by three months after surgery, it begins to grow in again at the normal rate of about one-half inch per month (figure C).

Four sessions are needed for punch graft transplantation. At the second session, which can be done three weeks after the first, additional plugs are transplanted between the original ones. Later, more grafts are transplanted between the rows of the first set.

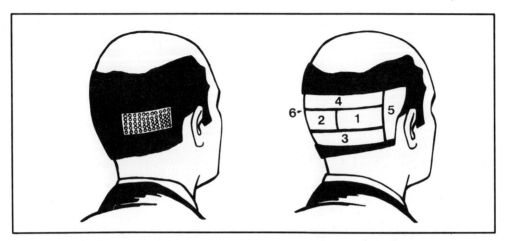

Punch grafts can be obtained from six different regions as shown here. The hair is trimmed only in the current donor site at the time of surgery. Approximately 60 grafts can be taken from each region. Some hair is left between each graft site to facilitate camouflaging.

Spacing of Grafts in Recipient Sites

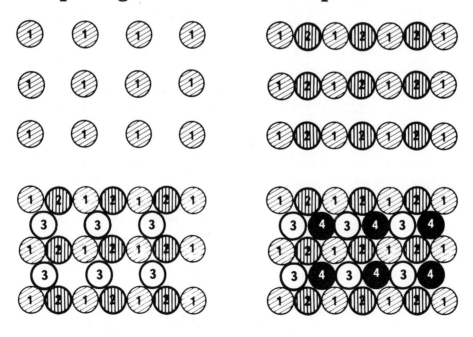

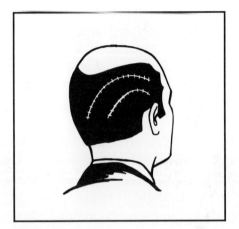

Figure D

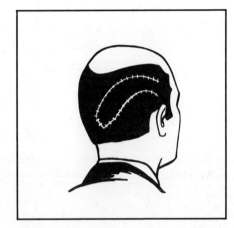

Figure E

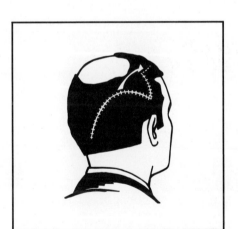

Figure F

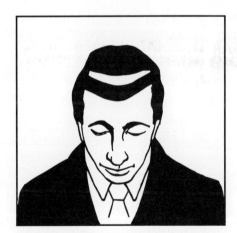

Figure G

The advantages? Punch graft transplantation is a relatively simple procedure that can be done under local anesthesia. Recovery time is minimal, and normal activities can be resumed quickly.

However, because of the way hair transplant grafts must be placed, normal density can never be achieved. Hair in the transplanted area grows in little tufts, similar to a doll's hair. The man must learn to style his hair carefully to camouflage this effect, and he must avoid getting his hair wet or windblown, which makes the tufting obvious. In addition, depending on the degree of baldness, punch grafts can take two to three years to complete.

It may now be possible to refine the hairline after hair transplantation surgery, explains the surgeon from California. The latest work in this area involves the use of micrografts or minigrafts—very small grafts of perhaps a single hair each are placed in the hairline to refine it and minimize the "corn-row" appearance. While minigrafts can't be done all over the head, the procedure gives a more natural hairline to hair transplant patients and eliminates some of the worry that the transplant will be noticed.

Scalp Flap Surgery

The newest means of hair replacement surgery, scalp flaps, can totally eliminate baldness for some people. Although it involves more radical surgery, the results are immediate—and dramatic. The front hairline is restored, and normal hair density is maintained.

To achieve this, large sections of hair-bearing scalp from the side and back of the head are loosened, rotated, and moved to the front of the head. The flaps are left attached at one end, so the hair is never totally separated from its blood supply. This means no temporary hair loss, a major drawback of the punch graft technique.

Two preliminary procedures are required in the surgeon's office before the actual surgery. First, the surgeon plans your new hairline with your cooperation, and he marks a four-centimeter (1-1/2 inch) wide strip on the side of your head, which is long enough to go across the entire bald spot to the fringe hair on the opposite side of your head. Then the

What Causes Baldness?

Scientists know that baldness has nothing to do with frequent shampooing or wearing a tight hat. Nor does the amount of oil in your skin, your skin type or complexion, or the amount of sun you get make any difference. The simple fact is that hair loss is something over which you have no control.

Heredity does play a role. If baldness runs in your family, you are likely to have a tendency toward baldness yourself. But any man may be the first in his family to lose his hair. And it's not uncommon for one man to enjoy a full head of hair while his brother goes bald.

Hormones are an important factor. Although scientists are not sure why, they know that baldness stops in men who have been surgically castrated (to treat cancer of the testicles, for example). Women can suffer hair loss also, although this is much more rare. Baldness also can be caused by burns, accidents, tumor surgery, radiation therapy, skin diseases, and some rare conditions.

surgeon makes an incision on each side of the strip along 80 percent of its length and stitches this incision closed (figure D). You wear a bandage overnight, which you may remove the next morning to resume most normal activities.

You return one week later to complete the process of separating the flap from its blood supply. The surgeon makes two more incisions at the lower end of the flap (figure E), stitches them closed, and applies a bandage. No hair is cut during either of these procedures.

After one more week, the actual flap transfer is performed. This may be done in a hospital or in an office surgery center, usually under general

Balloons Expand the Scalp

A new technique called tissue expansion can be used when the scalp is too tight for conventional scalp reduction. ''Skin will stretch as long as it is done slowly,'' says the facial plastic surgeon from California. ''Look at how it stretches to accommodate pregnancy.'' Ugandan women with their lower lips grossly extended over an inserted plate also are familiar with the skin's ability to expand.

In this procedure, the surgeon implants a deflated balloon under skin of the hair-bearing scalp. Twice a week, sterile water is injected into the balloon, stretching the skin slightly. A pulling feeling may be noted for a day or so, but then the skin relaxes. Injections continue over a period of six to eight weeks, until the desired expansion has been achieved. Then the balloon is removed, the bald area cut away, and the newly stretched hair-bearing scalp used to cover the area.

''Balloon expansion is used more commonly in reconstructive cases,'' says the surgeon from California. Most people, he adds, have enough looseness in the skin of their scalp to accommodate scalp reduction surgery. Patients who have suffered extensive hair loss due to burns, injury, or cancer surgery are more likely to need stretching, and are more accepting of the necessary inconvenience.

If you require tissue expansion, take along a large hat and a sense of humor.

or twilight anesthesia. A strip of bald scalp is removed, and the prepared strip of hair-bearing skin is rotated into position. The opening on the back or side of the head is closed by gently stretching the surrounding skin (figure F). The resulting scar is hidden by the hair.

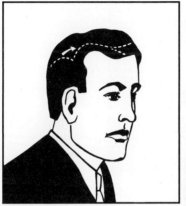

Figure H

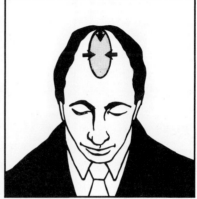

Figure I

You must wear a bandage for a couple of days and return to have stitches removed six days later, after which you may begin styling your hair. A minor touch-up procedure may be needed about six weeks later to remove a small flap of folded skin, called a dog ear, at the point where the scalp flap was rotated. If your baldness is extensive, a second flap can be moved from the opposite side of the head and placed in back of the first flap three months after the first surgery is completed (figure G).

Scalp flap surgery causes no change in the texture or density of your hair—whatever you have in back is exactly what you will get on top. The result is a more uniform, natural thickness of hair that can be styled conventionally. You can part your hair down the middle or climb out of a swimming pool without worry—no one will notice that you have had hair replacement surgery. The incision in your new hairline is finished in a way that allows hair to grow through the scar, camouflaging it very effectively.

Scalp flaps involve more extensive surgery and deeper anesthesia than punch grafts, but many men feel the difference in the results make the inconvenience worthwhile. The amount of discomfort is greater: "Doctors call this minor surgery, but I had some discomfort," David R. notes. "I experienced an anxiety period wondering whether it would work or not." Complications also are possible, although these are generally minor and correctable.

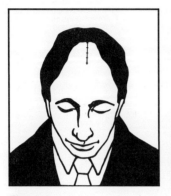

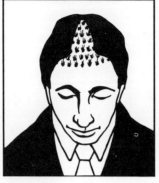

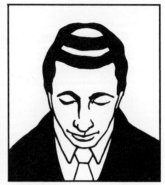

Figure J   *Figure K*   *Figure L*

Short Flaps

A similar but much less extensive procedure is possible for some individuals whose baldness is limited to the front of the head. The preliminary procedures are not necessary. A short flap, about one-inch wide and long enough to cover half the hairline, is moved to the front of the head (figure H). About three weeks later, a similar flap is moved forward from the opposite side of the head.

Candidates for this procedure must be chosen with extreme care. It is important to determine that baldness will not continue to progress, because once the short flap procedure has been done, it is not possible to do the more extensive scalp flap surgery at a later date.

Scalp Reduction Surgery

One of the latest techniques for reducing baldness is scalp reduction surgery. The surgeon actually decreases the size of the bald area by stretching and advancing the adjacent hair-bearing scalp and cutting out the bald area. This technique usually is used in conjunction with either scalp flap surgery or punch grafts.

''This procedure gives us a real advantage,'' explains the surgeon from Beverly Hills, Calif., ''because if the size of the bald area can be reduced, fewer punch grafts need to be used, and normal density can be maintained over a larger area of the scalp.''

Baldness—No Instant Panacea

Men have tried for centuries to find solutions to baldness. Success, however, has remained elusive. The most common solution for hair loss today is still the hairpiece. A high quality wig or hairpiece can give the appearance of a full head of hair instantly. But good quality hairpieces are expensive, and, over a lifetime, it may cost more to have several hairpieces made than to have hair replacement surgery. Hairpieces also require frequent cleaning, which may require the purchase of a second hairpiece to wear when the primary one is being cleaned.

A hairpiece that shifts or moves can cause embarrassment, so techniques for fixing it to the scalp have been developed. Adhesives probably are the safest method for fixing a hairpiece, but they can cause irritation and itching. Stitches or staples that actually attach the hairpiece to the scalp have been tried, but these have proven dangerous. Any foreign substance inserted into the scalp can cause severe infections, and some states have passed laws banning such procedures.

A less invasive procedure, "hair weaving," involves attaching a hairpiece with thread to existing hair. This method has serious disadvantages. Although secure at first, the hairpiece loosens as the hair grows and must be tightened every six to eight weeks. Ironically, hair weaving may actually cause further hair loss as the constant tension damages the remaining healthy hair.

What about minoxidil, the new drug that is said to grow hair? Minoxidil originally was introduced as a blood pressure medication. When it was found to cause hair growth on some patients, the news was received with great enthusiasm by those who hoped it might be the answer to curing baldness.

continued

Minoxidil taken internally does cause hair growth, but not necessarily on the head. When made into a lotion and rubbed on the scalp, hair growth does occur in some individuals, but not all—and for many the results may be thin, patchy, and not cosmetically appealing. It is not yet known how long the drug must be used to maintain hair growth, but early tests indicate that hair falls out if the drug is discontinued. The drug is very expensive, and long-term side effects are as yet unknown.

Research into the causes and cures of baldness continues, but many questions remain. Nothing is available today that can be taken internally or rubbed on the scalp that safely and reliably causes hair to grow for most individuals. A genuine cure for baldness would be known worldwide in just a few weeks. Therefore, when it comes to so-called baldness cures, let the buyer beware.

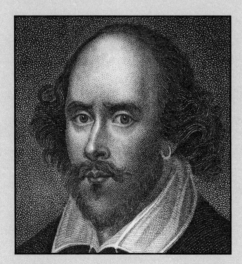

William Shakespeare had a problem with male pattern baldness; so, it is said, did Julius Caesar.

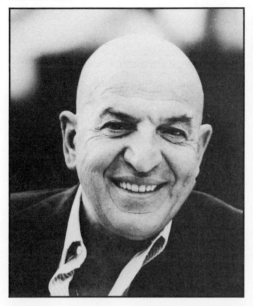 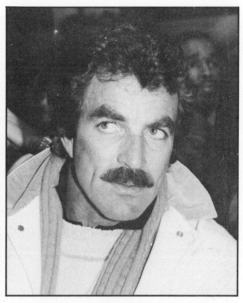

Sometimes hair counts, and sometimes it doesn't, as Telly Savalas and Tom Selleck plainly illustrate.

In this procedure, portions of the bald scalp are removed and the remainder of the scalp, including the hair-bearing areas, are stretched closed (figure I). This stretching does thin the hair-bearing scalp, but not significantly.

The patient may return to work the day after surgery with rare exceptions. Scalp reductions are office procedures that leave scars within the bald areas of the scalp. These are camouflaged by the surrounding hair or by punch grafting the remaining bald areas. Scalp reductions performed prior to punch grafting decrease the total area that must be covered (figures I, J, K).

Sometimes scalp reduction is done after scalp flap surgery to eliminate bald patches between the first and second flaps (figure L). For patients with only a small bald area on the crown, scalp reduction surgery may even totally eliminate the baldness.

Which procedure is best? Anyone who is a candidate for punch grafts also is a candidate for scalp flaps. Candidates for either procedure must have adequate donor hair for the surgery to be successful. Asking your-self the following questions might help you decide:

- Am I willing to undergo the more complex scalp flap surgery, or does the simplicity of punch grafts appeal to me more?
- How do I feel about deep anesthesia?
- How often am I outdoors in windy weather, in athletic contests that cause me to perspire, or in water—activities that may reveal punch grafts?

To Have or Not to Have Hair

Not everyone is a candidate for hair replacement surgery. First of all, you must have sufficient hair remaining to serve as a donor area. If your hair is very thin, you may have to accept your baldness or wear a conventional hairpiece. Second, your baldness pattern must be well es-tablished. If hair loss has just begun, you would be well advised to wait until the ultimate extent of your baldness can be accurately determined.

"The extent of baldness usually is predictable by the mid to late 20s," explains the surgeon from California, "and the size of the bald area is important in relation to the size of the donor area. When evaluating a patient, I assume that all of the thinning area is totally bald."

It can be tragic, he adds, to have hair replacement surgery done in-appropriately at too early an age. Transplanted hair can fall out if it was drawn from an area destined for eventual baldness. "I've seen patients who wanted me to repair damage done by early, poorly done transplant procedures," the surgeon explains. "Some have had all their donor hair used up and are left with with visible scars or abnormal patterns of bald-ness. These men are almost tearful when I tell them nothing can be done. They would take their natural baldness back in an instant, but it is al-ready too late."

As with any facial plastic surgery procedure, it is imperative to select a surgeon with experience in the technique and evidence of good prior results. A good surgeon takes the time to be certain that donor hair is permanent and determines before surgery what procedures should or should not be done. If done right, hair replacement surgery is a lifetime procedure. If it will not last a lifetime, it should not be done, the California facial plastic surgeon insists. To do otherwise is not ethical. "Surgeons who get the best results are the ones who take time to evaluate patients carefully beforehand," he says.

Physical factors are not the only considerations. Your motivation for having the surgery and your goals and expectations about the surgery must be discussed thoroughly. If you want hair replacement to fix your love life or guarantee a promotion, you are doing it for the wrong reasons. "Some people simply should not have surgery," the facial plastic surgeon from California explains.

Here are some questions you may be asked to help determine your motivation and expectations:

- Why do you want hair replacement surgery?
- Have you investigated or used another method of treatment for baldness? If yes, why were you dissatisfied with it?
- Why do you want hair replacement surgery now? How long have you been thinking about having this surgery done?
- Whose idea is it to have the surgery?
- What other surgical procedures have you had or would you like to have? Were you happy with the results of previous surgery?
- Have you ever been treated by a psychiatrist or psychologist?
- What do you think this procedure will do for you?
- Do you have any idea how you will look when the surgery is completed? What appearance will satisfy you?
- Do you understand that this procedure is designed to improve your appearance, not to achieve perfection?
- Do you understand that this procedure might not fully satisfy your expectations?

The cost of the procedure may or may not be a deciding factor to you. Cost depends on several factors, including the degree of hair loss and the procedures required. Generally, surgery costs little more than a good quality hairpiece for the same area. Depending on the complexity of the surgery, this can range from $2,000 to $20,000.

The Growing Popularity of Hair Replacement Surgery

Interest in hair replacement surgery is growing, facial plastic surgeons report. Like other types of facial plastic surgery, hair replacement can help you look better and feel better about yourself.

More men are having hair replacement surgery than you might think. Unlike women, who frequently are willing to talk about facelifts or other facial plastic surgery, men often don't like others to know that they have had hair replacement surgery. Many men just are not ready to admit that they care about their appearance to that extent.

However, men do care. Most men who have had hair replacement surgery are glad they did, according to a California facial plastic surgeon's survey. A majority reported feeling more self-confident after hair replacement surgery and said that their relationships with others had improved. Nearly two-thirds reported a significant rise in income after having had the surgery, presumably because of job advancement triggered by improved self-esteem.

Of course, not everyone feels as strongly about hair loss. Many men are content to let nature take its course. Yul Brenner and Telly Savalas have made their careers of a bald pate. But if looking older than you are is causing you to lose confidence in yourself; if baldness is a liability in your professional life; or if you feel young, active, and vigorous and want to look that way, hair replacement surgery may provide a practical alternative.

IV

Presenting the New You

19

Postoperative Skin Care and Cosmetic Tips

YOUR SURGERY IS COMPLETED, and your incisions have begun to heal. So why are you feeling depressed?

It is quite common to feel depressed during the first few days or weeks following surgery, warns a facial plastic surgeon from New Rochelle, N.Y. Final results are not yet visible, your face is bruised and swollen, and you are feeling drained from the surgery or the anesthesia. You are wondering, ''Why did I do this?''

It is natural to be anxious to see your new look. Just remember that facial plastic surgery is major surgery, and the healing process takes time. You should expect to feel fatigued or just rundown for a day or two after surgery. The tired feeling may continue for a week or more, depending on which procedures you have had.

''I didn't go to work for a week,'' recalls Marcia C. of Jacksonville, Fla., of her facelift surgery. ''Every morning I would get up and shower, then I would take my cotton swabs and go over the incisions with peroxide before applying ointment. I went for walks every day and had

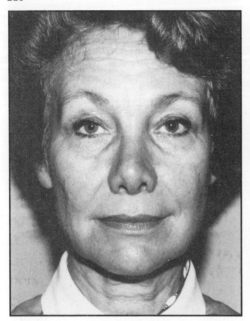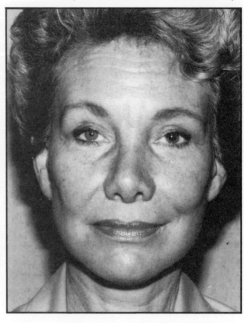

Gaye Collier was thoroughly pleased with the result of her facial plastic surgery.

a great time. I rested—just took it easy and felt like a queen for an entire week.''

Most patients report similar experiences. In fact, very few complain of significant postoperative pain. A recent survey conducted by the American Academy of Facial Plastic and Reconstructive Surgery reveals that 15 percent of facial plastic surgery patients report no discomfort at all while 58 percent experience minimal discomfort. Only 27 percent say they experienced actual pain.

What If Nobody Notices?

It bears repeating that the best facial plastic surgery is surgery that does not dramatically change your looks but, rather, effects more subtle change that makes you look rested and refreshed. Few individuals want results so dramatic that acquaintances stop them on the street to ask if

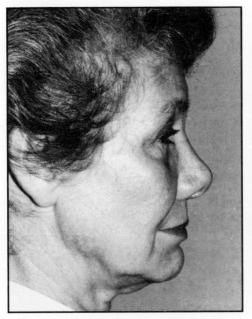 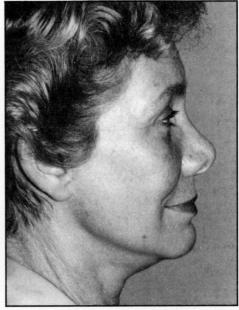

they have had facial plastic surgery. On the other hand, you may be dismayed if nobody notices a change at all.

There are several possible explanations for this. Often friends and colleagues will notice a change but are not certain if they should mention the improvement to respect your privacy. Sometimes an element of jealousy intervenes. Close friends actually may be envious of your new, improved look and may refrain from mentioning how good you look. Family members frequently have become so accustomed to seeing you with wrinkles or drooping skin or a large nose that they, in effect, don't see those imperfections at all. Thus, they may not notice when the imperfections are gone. This is why facial plastic surgeons are adamant that the patient's motivation for having the surgery come from within—from a desire for personal improvement, not to impress someone else. ''I did it for me,'' is the statement heard most often by satisfied facial plastic surgery patients.

When You Do Not Want the World to Know

Not everyone wants to tell the world that he or she has had facial plastic surgery, says Diane Young, a New York corrective cosmetic consultant. "I think it is important to have a strategy planned before you go back to work or appear in public."

Young advises drawing attention away from your face by making some other change in your appearance before surgery. For example, change your hairstyle. Make it straighter or curlier. Begin using clips or combs. Have it cut shorter. Change your hair color subtly by adding highlights, or use a product to cover gray. "This gives people something else to focus on besides your face," Young explains, "and diverts attention away from the other changes that occur."

After surgery, keep your makeup simple, concentrating on concealing your scars and discoloration. Until you are fully healed, avoid dramatic eye colors, turtlenecks, or large earrings. Instead, Young advises, call attention away from your face with an upswept hairdo, a new hair color, an eye-catching bracelet, an attractive tie, or a pretty pin on on your blouse or lapel.

By drawing people's eyes away from your face, you can minimize the possibility that your scars will be noticed and ensure that your grand entrance will be a big success.

Give Yourself Time to Heal

You can expect to resume your normal activities about two weeks after surgery. In the interim, take care to protect your incisions and any swollen or reddened areas. Sleep with your head elevated during those first two weeks—and sleep alone to avoid being accidentally bumped by a sleeping partner. Do not pick up small children or heavy packages.

Cool compresses or ice will help reduce swelling as will staying quietly active. Be sure to rest when you feel tired, however. Avoid foods that require strenuous chewing, like corn on the cob, that might put stress on stitches. And do not get involved in any arguments or spirited discussions: Exaggerated facial movements may strain your incisions.

If you have had a facelift or neck surgery, avoid turning your head from side to side. Instead, rotate your head and shoulders as one unit. After a rhinoplasty, keep a stiff upper lip and avoid excess smiling. Don't blow your nose at all for the first 10 days, and then blow carefully through both sides at once.

Following dermabrasion or chemical peeling, use warm compresses to soothe the area and be sure to stay out of the sun during the first six months. Wear a wide-brimmed hat and sunglasses, stay in the shade whenever possible, and use a good sunblock (SPF 15 or higher) if you are going to be outside for any length of time. Avoid anything that dries your skin, like heat, cold, and wind, and use a moisturizer regularly.

Do not use aspirin or any aspirin-containing product, which inhibits blood clotting, for a period of from two weeks before your surgery to two weeks after, and avoid alcohol and smoking during this four-week period as well.

Refrain from bending and heavy lifting during the first two weeks after surgery. These activities may aggravate swelling, increase your blood pressure and cause you to start bleeding. You should wait three to six weeks before resuming such activities as aerobics, tennis, weightlifting, contact sports, and swimming or diving. Ask your facial plastic surgeon for specific advice about any of these activities.

"The main thing is to follow your doctor's advice," asserts Marcia. "Don't get frightened if at first you look a little different. Just keep an ice bag on, elevate your head, and follow the doctor's orders."

Looking Your Best After Surgery

You can do quite a bit to promote rapid healing, lift your spirits, and enhance the results of your surgery. Many women enjoy having a professional consultation with a cosmetologist at this point. The facial plastic surgeon from New York supports this idea. "A positive attitude is essential, and proper use of cosmetics can do wonders for a patient's self-esteem," he says. "We can't eliminate bruising and swelling, but there is no reason why you can't look good shortly after surgery."

A variety of special cosmetics is available to help camouflage the inevitable swelling and bruising. Some surgeons carry such products in their offices and have trained staff members to help their patients achieve the look they want. Others refer their patients to nearby cosmetic consultants. "I urge all my patients to arrange a consultation at a salon that specializes in postoperative cosmetic care," the surgeon from New York says. "The patients love it. It is a truly great experience for them."

Skin Care is Important

"We find that people are happier with the results of their surgery if they go into it with skin that is in good condition," says Diane Young, whose facial care salon in New York City treats many of the above surgeon's patients. "Surgery traumatizes your skin and can cause temporary changes in the way it feels. Skin that is very oily or very dry tends to be worse after surgery."

Young recommends a deep-cleansing facial before any facial plastic surgery procedure. This will open pores and add moisture to the skin. "You should make sure that your skin is as healthy as possible before having surgery," she advises. To do this, abstain from smoking, aspirin, and alcohol, and avoid suntan parlors before surgery.

Neutralize Those Bruises

"The best way to cover bruises or large discolorations," says Diane Young, "is with an underbase skin toner." Toners, available in green, yellow, and purple, go on under the concealer to neutralize skin discolorations. "Using a small amount of underbase allows you to use less heavy concealer," Young explains. "You get a more natural look with less makeup."

Bruises generally go through several color changes, notes Young. The opposite color toner neutralizes the discoloration. For example:

- To cover excess redness, such as after a chemical peel or dermabrasion, use a green underbase.
- On purple bruises, use a yellow underbase.
- When the bruise turns yellow, use a purple underbase.

Over the toner, apply a concealer that matches your natural skin tone. Pat the concealer on over the discolored areas with light touch. This totally covers any discolorations, including freckles and other blemishes.

Several lines of concealing cosmetic products are available for facial plastic surgery patients. Specifically formulated to cover discoloration, the cosmetics are hypo-allergenic and contain a sunscreen. Since these products may not be available at your favorite cosmetic counter, ask your surgeon for more information on how to order the products you need.

Proper hygiene after surgery is essential to promote better healing. Every surgeon has an individual set of specific instructions for postsurgical skin care. In general, you must keep your incisions clean and dry and your skin properly moisturized. Follow your doctor's instructions to the letter for optimum healing.

Within two weeks after most facial plastic surgery procedures, the incisions are closed, crusts are coming off, the worst of the swelling has subsided, and you are ready to return to your normal routine. But do not go back to your old cosmetics just yet. Check with your surgeon about what kind of makeup you may use. Postsurgical cosmetics should be gentle to your skin but give you the coverage you need to camouflage your bruises.

Using Cosmetics After Surgery

How you will look two weeks after surgery will depend on what surgical procedures you have had and how quickly your own body heals. "We've seen people who come in with very deep bruises," says Diane Young. "Other people have only a tiny bit of discoloration. Everyone heals differently."

No matter how you look, as soon as your doctor gives the green light to wearing makeup, you can be made to look presentable. It makes no difference if you are a man or a woman. A variety of high-coverage corrective cosmetics is available for both men and women with special needs. These products effectively camouflage scars, bruises, burns, and untreatable birthmarks and other defects.

Most individuals can wear makeup about one week after surgery and 10 days after dermabrasion or chemical peeling. Ask your doctor when it is safe to start. Many surgeons recommend water-based cosmetics at first, since they can be easily washed off if irritation occurs. You may be advised to use cosmetics that are hypo-allergenic. Avoid products that contain fragrance or alcohol during the first few months.

Make sure that everything that comes in contact with your face is totally sanitary. Use cotton swabs, cotton balls, and disposable sponges instead of cosmetic brushes. Apply cosmetics carefully to avoid pulling or manipulating the skin.

Certain imperfections require special treatment as follows:

- *Scars.* Most incision scars from facial plastic surgery procedures are hidden and do not present a cosmetic problem. If there are noticeable scars, they can present problems if they are a different color than the surrounding skin, have a different texture, or are slightly raised or lowered. Color and texture problems are easily solved by using a foundation makeup with good coverage. Surface irregularities are more difficult to camouflage because they create shadows that do not mask easily. Avoid trying to cover a raised or depressed scar with makeup. Makeup tends to collect in slight depressions or along the edges of raised scars, making the blemish even more noticeable. Instead, use a sheer foundation up to the edges of the scar and play up your other features to draw the eye away from the irregularity. If the scar doesn't even out with time, check with your surgeon to see if dermabrasion might help.

- *Rhinoplasty.* It will take several months or even a year for all the swelling to recede and your nose to take its final shape. If you have had a prominent nose all your life, you will discover that when your nose is less prominent, your eyes assume more importance, so play up your eyes and make them your dominant feature. Be sure your eyebrows are well shaped, and use eye shadow colors that enhance your natural skin tone. Line your eyes only under your lower lashes—never on the inside rim of the eyes. Use a soft eyeliner pencil that won't pull the delicate skin of the eye area.

- *Eyelid surgery.* You will have a red incision line on your eyelid for a while. Dab on a little underbase with a green tint, then use concealer and powder your lids before applying eyelid color. If you have redness, avoid pink, purple, and brown eye shadow; use blue, gray, or blue-green instead. Use mascara that is formulated for sensitive eyes, and never keep it longer than six months.

After a facelift, choose a soft, face-framing hairdo. Hair that is too short around the face and hair that is swept up off the forehead may reveal scars. Medium-length bangs, perhaps gently curled, can help camouflage scars in the forehead area.

- If hairline and forehead scars are not a problem, a soft, full back-swept hairstyle can promote a youthful appearance. Avoid severely pulled back styles.

- If you have a reddened complexion or redness around your eyes, never wear fuschia, rose, red, or hot pink makeup colors. Instead, choose soft shades of blue and green for both your wardrobe and makeup.

Is Facial Plastic Surgery Worth It?

Ask almost anyone who has had facial plastic surgery, and most likely you will hear a resounding "yes!"

"It was a very pleasant experience," Marcia C. notes. "I'm not a vain person, but I do like to look my best. What this did was give me a little extra 'oomph' as far as confidence is concerned."

Marcia continues, as others have noted, that her colleagues at work did not realize she had had surgery. "Most thought I looked like I had been away on a month's vacation, because I seemed so relaxed and rested."

Perhaps the best indication of satisfaction is the high number of patients who say they would do it again—95 percent, according to a recent survey. Representative of those satisfied patients is Bob Damkroger: "I've had nasal surgery, an upper and lower blepharoplasty [eyelid surgery], and a full facelift. I'm going to have a chemical peel this fall to take away the crow's feet. I believe in looking as good as I can for as long as I can."

Looking good and feeling great. That is what facial plastic surgery is all about.

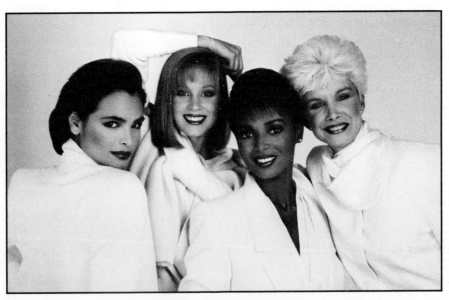

The correct color makeup can enhance the most beautiful face.

Some Additional Makeup Tips

- Some experts recommend using a foundation one shade lighter than your natural skin tone. Use a translucent powder after foundation for complete coverage with a soft, natural look.
- A concealer (stick or cream) may be applied under your eyes to mask bruises or dark circles. Apply it under your foundation, and use a shade slightly lighter than your base color.
- Scars in the eyebrow area may result in missing eyebrow hairs. Use a small, angled brush to shade the missing area with a flat eye shadow color close to your hair color. This looks more natural than shading with an eyebrow pencil.
- A soft eye shadow pencil in slate or taupe can be smudged toward the outer corner of the eye to correct any visible scars in this area.

- *Facelift.* Apply a neutralizing underbase and a concealer to the bruised areas. Then apply a thin coat of foundation in a shade that matches your natural skin tone as closely as possible, and blend carefully for a smooth, natural appearance.

Color Magic

Everyone's skin coloring fits into one of two basic categories—pink/blue or yellow/green. So says Diane Young, who explains that people with pink/blue skin tones should draw their makeup and hair coloring from the cool color family, and those with yellow/green skin tones should choose warm or earthy makeup colors.

Young's specific makeup tips:

Pink/blue Skin Tones:
- *Blush colors*—pink, rose, or red with blue undertones.
- *Lipstick shades*—pink, rose, plum, berry, clear red, or red with blue undertones.
- *Eye shadow*—neutral shades are taupe, gray, and navy; colors are any shade of pink and rose, blue, teal, lavender, plum, violet, or purple.

Yellow/green Skin Tones:
- *Blush colors*—earth tones like peach, bronze, cinnamon, or apricot.
- *Lipstick shades*—coral, apricot, bronze, peach, red with orange undertones, or orange.
- *Eye shadow*—neutral shades are cream, brown, and taupe; colors are all shades of green, gold, brown, peach, copper, apricot, bronze, and teal.

If you are over 25, your daytime eye colors should have no iridescence in them. Frosted eye shadows emphasise the tiny lines and wrinkles we all get as we grow older.

About the American Academy of Facial Plastic and Reconstructive Surgery

The American Academy of Facial Plastic and Reconstructive Surgery, an international medical society of more than 3,100 facial plastic surgeons, is the largest association of specialty plastic surgeons in the world. Membership is open to otolaryngologists-head and neck surgeons, dermatologists, ophthalmologists, general plastic surgeons, and other surgeons who are certified by an American examining board of specialists or its equivalent, and have training and experience in facial plastic surgery.

Academy fellows, as stipulated in the bylaws, must be fellows of the American College of Surgeons or its equivalent, and citizens or residents of the United States or Canada. They must have been actively engaged in practicing facial surgery for a period of three years prior to application, and they must submit a detailed report of 35 major facial plastic and reconstructive surgical procedures performed within a 12-month period in accordance with the criteria for such procedures established by the Academy board of directors.

The Academy promotes the study, research, and scientific advancement of facial plastic and reconstructive surgery and all related basic sciences. It is devoted to expanding the knowledge and improving the skills of facial plastic surgeons and the training of residents and other young physicians interested in this specialty.

The Academy's program of continuing medical education is widely respected by the medical community. Since it was established in 1964, the AAFPRS has been and is dedicated to the dissemination of knowledge. Its program of courses includes more than 35 seminars and workshops on all major aspects of facial plastic and reconstructive surgery. Its graduate fellowship program represents one of the finest opportunities for the education of facial plastic surgeons in the nation. Two relatively new programs—the observational education program and the visiting professors program—give members the opportunity to observe selected senior Academy fellows in their own operating rooms and offices, and senior members share their knowledge with residents in university hospital settings. In addition, an outstanding videotape series gives all members the opportunity to view the techniques of senior members. An awards program each year recognizes clinical or research-oriented contributions to the field. Several research grants are made each year.

Supplemental Information

The American Academy of Facial Plastic and Reconstructive Surgery publishes two additional sources of information that supplement this book—brochures and a quarterly newsletter. If you would like to receive either, simply complete and return the order form on the following page.

BROCHURES

The Academy's brochures were written by facial plastic surgeons and are available in Spanish as well as English. Each brochure describes in detail the problem or condition for which help is sought, the surgical treatment, the risks, costs, where surgery takes place, what kind of anesthesia is required, and so on.

[ ] YES, I'd like to receive the brochure(s) checked below. I understand no cost is involved.

[ ] Plastic Surgery of the Eyelids, Eyebrows, and Forehead

[ ] Plastic Surgery of the Nose

[ ] Facelift

[ ] Plastic Surgery of the Ear

[ ] Surgical Treatment of Facial Skin Blemishes

[ ] Surgical Treatment of Hair Loss

[ ] Facial Plastic Surgery

[ ] Dermabrasion

[ ] Facial Scar Revision

[ ] Postoperative Facial Skin Care and Cosmetic Tips

[ ] Plastic Surgery of the Chin

[ ] Facial Liposuction

[ ] Chemical Peeling

PATIENT NEWSLETTER

The Academy's patient newsletter, *Facial Plastic Surgery Today*, regularly features case studies of procedures and "before and after" photos. It covers scientific advances such as laser surgery and injectable fillers that offer new avenues for patient care. It reports cosmetic tips for different eye shapes, postoperative grooming, and hairstyles for variously shaped faces. The four-page, two-color newsletter is published quarterly.

How to Order

[ ] YES, I'd like to subscribe to the quarterly newsletter, *Facial Plastic Surgery Today*. I understand that there is no charge.

Name_____

Street_____ Address_____

City _____ State_____ Zip_____

PLEASE RETURN TO:
American Academy of Facial Plastic
and Reconstructive Surgery
1101 Vermont Ave. N.W., Suite 404
Washington, D.C. 20005

To place orders for brochures and the patient newsletter or to secure a list of AAFPRS fellows in your area, who have chosen to participate in the Facial Plastic Surgery Information Service, Inc., you may call toll-free 800-332-FACE (U.S.), 800-523-FACE (Canada), or 842-4500 (District of Columbia).